SPORTS AND ATHLETICS PREPARATION, PERFORMANCE, AND PSYCHOLOGY

EXERCISE TRAINING

TYPES AND METHODS, ROLE IN DISEASE PREVENTION AND HEALTH BENEFITS

SPORTS AND ATHLETICS PREPARATION, PERFORMANCE, AND PSYCHOLOGY

Additional books in this series can be found on Nova's website under the Series tab.

Additional e-books in this series can be found on Nova's website under the e-book tab.

SPORTS AND ATHLETICS PREPARATION, PERFORMANCE, AND PSYCHOLOGY

EXERCISE TRAINING

TYPES AND METHODS, ROLE IN DISEASE PREVENTION AND HEALTH BENEFITS

LUCY DUKES
EDITOR

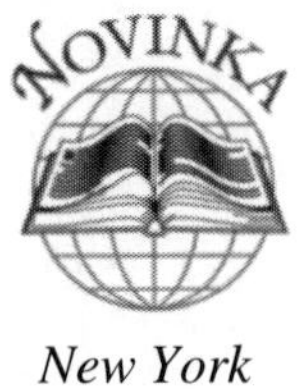

New York

For permission to use material from this book please contact us:
Telephone 631-231-7269; Fax 631-231-8175
Web Site: http://www.novapublishers.com

Library of Congress Cataloging-in-Publication Data

ISBN: 978-1-63463-501-1

Published by Nova Science Publishers, Inc. † New York

CONTENTS

PREFACE

Exercise is one component of daily energy expenditure in humans. It has become an important part of healthy lifestyles, because individuals are less active both at work and at home compared to earlier days and because today's environment makes it easy for individuals to be inactive, such as when people use elevators instead of stairs, cars instead of bicycles, and technology instead of activities with full body movement. This book discusses the types and methods of exercise training, as well as the role it plays in disease prevention.

Chapter 1 - Stroke was reported to be the second leading cause of death and the first leading cause of long-term disability in developed nations. It entails compromised brain function following a disturbance in local blood supply. Survivors of stroke present with persistent neurological defects manifested physically, emotionally, and mentally. Despite immense research, limited therapies exist. Exercise has long been known to provide neuroprotection to ischemic tissue and to improve prognosis of stroke. Early exercise in particular seems to confer neuroplasticity following stroke, mediated by mechanisms such as neurogenesis, angiogenesis, and synaptogenesis. The cause for contention, however, is determining the ideal window of opportunity to maximize the benefits from exercise therapy and minimizing the potential for secondary complications. This article seeks to shed light on some contemporary exercise-mediated therapies and the variables involved. Variables under investigation that could potentially improve prognosis in stroke patients include exercise onset, type, and intensity. Special attention is allocated to eliciting the effects of early exercise at the cellular and molecular levels with the use of human studies as well as animal models.

Chapter 2 - The goal of this chapter is to review the importance of contextual exercise factors, such as a certain name of exercise bouts (e.g., "fat-burning") and a certain framing of exercise bouts (e.g., "enjoyable activity"), for food consumption depending on consumers' goal states. In an effort to follow a healthy lifestyle, individuals have various goals in mind. These goals are often incompatible to each other and therefore produce goal conflicts in individuals, such as the conflict between wanting to watch a movie with friends in the evening and wanting a fit body. Against the background of the increasing prevalence of overweight and obesity worldwide, this chapter specifically looks at goal conflicts of individuals that are at greatest risk of failing to achieve their long-term goals, such as self-imposed exercisers or dietary restrained eaters, and presents empirical evidence that contextual exercise references often rather harm (than help) vulnerable consumer groups attain desirable long-term health and fitness goals. The chapter discusses implications from the perspective of public health and product/service providers.

Chapter 3 - The social and economic transformations which society has undergone since the last century have caused significant changes in morbidity and mortality in our population profile. Infectious and parasitic diseases, the leading causes of death in the beginning of last century, gave way to Chronic Non-Communicable Diseases (CNCDs). In 2008, the CNCDs were responsible for 63% of those occurring in the world and approximately 80% of these occur in low and middle income. The main causes of these diseases include modifiable risk factors such as smoking, harmful alcohol consumption, physical inactivity and unhealthy diet, and non-modifiable factors such as age, heredity, gender and race. Anti-inflammatory effects by reducing systemic levels of proinflammatory adipokines and changes in markers inflammation via the production of IL-6. Plasma levels of IL-6 increase exponentially during physical exercise and greater stimuli for its synthesis appears to be related to the decrease of glycogen content in muscle. Increased levels of intracellular calcium and increased formation of reactive oxygen species are also capable of activating the transcription factors that regulate the synthesis of IL-6. This increase in circulating IL-6 is responsible for a subsequent increase of circulating anti-inflammatory cytokines. Furthermore, most of these anti-inflammatory effects are secondary to decreased concentration of triglycerides in plasma and low density lipoprotein (LDL) and increasing the concentration of high density lipoprotein (HDL) generated by improved lipid profile induced by exercise, and another beneficial response to exercise is the syntax stimulation of endothelial nitric oxide. Research clearly demonstrate the effectiveness of exercise in preventing diseases, especially cardiovascular, thus increasing levels of physical activity has been shown to decrease mortality and all the different diseases worldwide causes. The guide recognizes the benefits of cardiovascular disease prevention, and encourages the promotion of health, wellness and fitness to the public in order to improve the overall quality of life of individuals. Research is need on the potential benefits of differential training as an approach to physical rehabilitation and exercise prescription could counteract the psychological effects of physical disease in different populations.

Chapter 4 - The pineal gland is responsible for the synthesis and secretion of the hormone melatonin, which, in turn, participates in the temporal organization of biological rhythms acting as a mediator between the light / dark cycle and regulatory physiological processes, including the regulation of the cardiovascular system, immune system and, among others, the energy metabolism, influencing the secretion and action of insulin and increasing the thermogenic capacity of brown adipose tissue and the browning process. Moreover, melatonin presents powerful antioxidant, neuroprotective and neurogenic actions. The available data shows that melatonin is essential for adipose and muscle tissues metabolic adaptations to aerobic training. On the other hand, exercise training plays a key role in the control of glycemia, blood pressure, adult neurogenesis and browning of white adipose tissue. The reduction of melatonin production that occurs during aging, in diabetes, during shift-work or at illuminated environments during the night, not only impairs the metabolic benefits of exercise training but also induces several metabolic disorders such as insulin resistance, glucose intolerance, obesity and cardiovascular disturbances. Considering the available scientific evidence, clinicians may consider melatonin replacement or supplementation in certain situations, as the ones mentioned above, as an additional therapeutic tool in order to favor all the beneficial effects of the physical training.

In: Exercise Training
Editor: Lucy Dukes

ISBN: 978-1-63463-501-1

Chapter 1

EFFECTS OF PHYSICAL EXERCISE FOLLOWING ISCHEMIC STROKE: IS TIMING AN IMPORTANT FACTOR?

Fauzia Akbary, MSc[1,*], Krzysztof Grzegorczyk, HBSc[2,†] and Yuchuan Ding, MD, MSc, PhD[3,‡]

[1]Wayne State University School of Medicine, Detroit, MI, US
[2]University of Toronto, Toronto, Ontario, Canada
[3]Wayne State University School of Medicine, Department of Neurosurgery, Detroit, MI, US

ABSTRACT

Stroke was reported to be the second leading cause of death and the first leading cause of long-term disability in developed nations. It entails compromised brain function following a disturbance in local blood supply. Survivors of stroke present with persistent neurological defects manifested physically, emotionally, and mentally. Despite immense research, limited therapies exist. Exercise has long been known to provide

* Fauzia Akbary, MSc: Wayne State University School of Medicine. E-mail: fakbary@med.wayne.edu.

† Krzysztof Grzegorczyk, HBSc: University of Toronto. E-mail: krzysztof.grzegorczyk@utoronto.ca.

‡ Dr. Yuchuan Ding, MD, MSc, PhD: Wayne State University School of Medicine, Department of Neurosurgery. E-mail: yding@med.wayne.edu.

neuroprotection to ischemic tissue and to improve prognosis of stroke. Early exercise in particular seems to confer neuroplasticity following stroke, mediated by mechanisms such as neurogenesis, angiogenesis, and synaptogenesis. The cause for contention, however, is determining the ideal window of opportunity to maximize the benefits from exercise therapy and minimizing the potential for secondary complications. This article seeks to shed light on some contemporary exercise-mediated therapies and the variables involved. Variables under investigation that could potentially improve prognosis in stroke patients include exercise onset, type, and intensity. Special attention is allocated to eliciting the effects of early exercise at the cellular and molecular levels with the use of human studies as well as animal models.

INTRODUCTION

Stroke is a major cause of disability and death in developed countries [1] ranking second to ischemic heart disease [2]. Surviving stroke patients present with persistent neurological defects manifested physically, emotionally, and mentally. Approximately 85% of stroke patients experience complications at the hospital, and more than half of them die as a result of complications stemming from immobility [3]. Additionally, 1/3 of patients will die from recurrent stroke within 12 months of the initial stroke, while another 1/3 will be restricted to the most basic activities of daily living (ADL) [4].

Despite immense research, limited neuro-therapies exist.

However, the potential of exercise-mediated therapy for functional recovery post-stroke is well-recognized. Exercise exacts many health benefits and shows promise in providing neuroprotection to ischemic tissue. In fact, exercise therapy is currently widely administered to post-stroke patients. Benefits of exercise in older adults, a population more vulnerable to stroke, include increased chances of survival and healthier ageing in general [5].

Additionally, studies show that training or rehabilitation induces neuroplasticity in regions surrounding the lesion site and the contralateral hemisphere [6]. Despite the prevalence of its use in therapy for stroke patients, an optimal rehabilitation method for stroke patients pertaining to exercise onset, dose intensity, and type remains to be fully characterized [7]. Although clinical research strongly supports early mobilization and training [8], some studies have demonstrated that early exercise may not be beneficial but rather exacerbate brain damage following focal brain ischemia [9-11].

Therein lies the dilemma: how early is early exercise onset in order to be deemed maximally therapeutic to stroke survivors. This review article seeks to discuss the rehabilitative capacity of early exercise in stroke patients, to navigate through the current debate pertaining to defining early in early exercise, and the potential molecular and physiological basis underlying the exercise-mediated rehabilitation post-stroke.

EXERCISE REHABILITATION TODAY

Rehabilitation today recognize that as many as 50-70% of stroke survivors suffer from motor impairments and disabilities such as muscle weakness, reduced mobility, loss of strength and dexterity, and the inability to maintain balance [12, 13]. In reflection, the aims of rehabilitation therapy enable patients to enjoy an adequate quality of life by restoring sufficient function to allow patients to perform the ADL thus maintaining a continued sense of independence [14].

Current Models of Exercise-Mediated Recovery in Clinical Setting

To achieve the most positive outcome, patients are admitted to a stroke unit as early as possible. These units stabilize the patient's medical condition, develop the optimal treatment plan, make efforts to reduce the overall death rate, and to reduce the time spent in the hospital [15]. Once stabilized, rehabilitation becomes the main focus. This process often begins 1-2 days following stroke, taking place either at an in-patient or out-patient facility, or is home-based--all of which occur under the supervision and counsel of a team of physiotherapists, psychologists, occupation therapists, and psychologists. The rehabilitative process comprises of two phases: the early acute phase and the late phase. The early acute phase is essential in reducing secondary complications and impairments while promoting independence. In the late phase, the focus shifts to preventing secondary stroke [16]. However, no process coincides without its challenges. Although contemporary rehabilitative models focus on the acute stroke period primarily to facilitate ADL and functional recovery [17], many patients stop therapy prematurely and are discharged without achieving full recovery. Consequently, almost half of these patients regress in functional mobility within a year [18].

There are many hurdles associated with identifying the optimal rehabilitative strategy for stroke patients. One such factor is the patients' poor capacity for exercise [19, 20]. These patients exert as little as 40% of the capacity of age- and gender-matched individuals with a sedentary lifestyle [21, 22]. Meanwhile, the energy requirements of these patients with hemiparetic gait is increased by 55-100% [23, 24]. Energy requirements may be even greater in patients with neurological disability due to biomechanical inefficiency. Additionally, these individuals have low endurance which can further limit their mobility [17, 23, 25, 26]. In a 50-yard ambulation task, stroke patients experienced dyspnea, progressive slowing, and reduced motor dexterity. Meanwhile, chronic stroke patients exhibited VO2 levels half that of control individuals, levels which were only sufficient for performing basic ADL. Consequently, performing middle or upper range ADL was exhausting and often impossible. Henceforth, achieving even small gains in fitness levels translates to significant functional gains in stroke patients.

This marks the premise for developing exercise interventions of adequate duration and intensity with the correct onset to stimulate peak aerobic fitness and to facilitate recovery [22].

Clinical Evidence-Based Effects of Early Exercise on Stroke Outcome

For patients with mild to moderate disability following stroke, an early exercise intervention has shown to be one of the most effective forms of rehabilitation [27]. A large meta-review of 21 studies published by Ada et al. concluded that progressive resistance exercise <6 months post-stroke led to significant improvement in patient strength as well as level of activity. Meanwhile, only some improvements ensued in patients in the chronic phase (>6 months). It is thought that the observed difference can be attributed to a greater loss in muscle strength incurred from reduced muscle use and motor unit activity during the chronic phase [28]. This finding poses the important question of whether starting exercise rehabilitation even earlier will lead to an even better stroke outcome.

Overwhelming evidence from clinical studies indicates that exercise initiated within 30 days post-stroke leads to improved functional recovery [19]. In a study of 364 hemorrhagic stroke patients, those admitted to a rehabilitation program within 24 hours of admission performed much better on the Fugl-Myer Assessment Scale (FMA) and Modified Barthel Index (MBI) compared to their control counterparts who received standard hospital ward and internal medical treatment. The most significant gains were observed within the first month [20].

Additional evidence supporting this supposition comes from one of the first large-scale clinical studies looking at the effects of early exercise rehabilitation, AVERT (A Very Early Rehabilitation Trial). This study indicated that patients admitted to a rehabilitative program within 24 hours of stroke onset exhibited positive outcomes. Patients in both the intervention and control group were mobilized out of bed on an average of 18.1 hours and 30.8 hours, respectively, post-stroke with intensity—frequency, length, and level of activity—higher in the intervention group. Their rehabilitative therapy comprised of 10 activities including lying, activities in bed, supported sit, sitting activities, sit-to-stand, standing, early gait, advanced gait, upper-limb training, and other. Both groups received the same baseline standard care. There was no correlation between therapy dose or frequency and the number of adverse events 3 months post-stroke [29].

An additional difference observed between the two groups lay in the capacity of these patients to walk 50m unassisted: the interventional group was able to walk 50m unassisted significantly faster (3.5 days) than the standard care group (7.0 days). Furthermore, Barthel Index and Rivermead Motor Assessment measured at 3 months post-stroke associated the interventional group to better functional outcome [30].

A second study known as the Very Early Rehabilitation of Intensive Telemetry After Stroke (VERITAS) exhibited similar dramatic results when using the same protocol as AVERT (with respect to timing, nature and frequency of intervention) to treat the intervention group. Within 5 days of admission, 74% of the patients in the early mobilization group were able to walk independently, compared to 44% in the standard care group. The former group also exhibited a trend of achieving independence by 3 months with fewer medical complications after adjusting for age and stroke severity [31]. By amalgamating findings from both AVERT and VERITAS, the onset of initial mobilization post-stroke was significantly shorter (21 hrs) in the intervention group compared to its standard care counterpart (31 hrs). The early mobilization onset patients also exhibited a greater chance of acquiring independence by 3 months [31].

An additional study supporting early rehabilitation post-stroke comes from the Post-Stroke Rehabilitation Outcomes Project (PSROP) which looked at 1291 patients in six inpatient rehabilitation facilities. Findings indicated that delaying admission upon onset of stroke, moderate and severe, resulted in lower discharge functional independence (FIM) scores and increased length of stay (LOS). Consequently, the delay time between stroke onset and admission is a significant predictor of discharge total FIM score, discharge motor FIM score, discharge mobility FIM score, and rehabilitation LOS. The greatest gains in improved functional outcome were observed in the subgroup with the most severe stroke [32].

Aerobic exercise has been shown to have significant therapeutic effects in mild and moderately-impaired stroke patients [12]. It can include activities such as rowing, cycling, running, walking, and stepping. For patients with impaired balance, a stationary bike is used.

Patients unable to bear weight on an affected paretic leg are often engaged in aerobic water exercise, which provides some weight support, reducing joint impact loading, while still offering sufficient resistance [12].

A large meta-review of 151 studies published by van Peppen et al., found that the greatest therapeutic outcomes are from a combination of direct, focused tasks of sufficient intensity and early onset [27].

In summary, the discussed studies posit support for a strong association between early enrollment into a physical activity/exercise-based rehabilitation program and improved functional outcome following stroke. In addition, very early mobilization has shown to reduce medical complications as well as the time necessary to restore functional walking capacity. Similar to early mobilization, late rehabilitation is also somewhat associated with better stroke outcome [28]. It is important to note, however, that clinical studies have many limitations and possible confounding variables. There is very limited data with regards to early exercise effects on patients with more severe stroke, as well as for all stroke patients undergoing exercise immediately following stroke onset (<18 hrs). Similarly, some very early mobilization studies have reached inconclusive results [33]. Furthermore, despite very early exercise generally being promoted [34], it remains somewhat controversial [35, 36]. With the use of animal models such as the well-established rat stroke model, it is much easier to control for variables such as stroke severity or precise location of infarct and to study much earlier exercise onset.

Effects of Late Exercise and Other Factors in a Clinical Setting

In a human clinical study applying learning-based sensorimotor training (LBSMT) beginning 6 months after stroke, improvements ensued with respect to patient independence, fine motor skills, sensory discrimination, and strength. LBSMT is a neuroplasticity-based approach comprised of progression through a set of tasks related to discriminating shapes and textures, vibrations and force, controlling force, holding and eventually moving objects all with the affected hand [15]. After 6-8 weeks, patients that were subject to great intensity of training (i.e. frequency and duration) had much better outcome than their control counterparts who experienced training of lower intensity [37]. Although late exercise is indicated to be effective in maintaining and even improving function and independence through intense LBSMT in stroke patients [37], there is an ever increasing evidence for early and intensive activity to facilitate and accelerate return to unassisted walking and functional recovery in stroke patients [30].

Depending on the onset of late exercise, human studies in general have concluded that brain injury patients can indeed reap the benefits from a late exercise regimen, although such benefits are not as great as if the exercise was started early. Additionally, delaying rehabilitation significantly increases the risks of medical complications [3]. A study supporting late exercise demonstrated that functional benefits in the late stage of recovery post-stroke do ensue learning-based therapy. Additionally, LBSMT for 6-8 weeks was associated with a non-linear positive correlation between training intensity (measured by frequency of weekly visits) and motor functional recovery [37].

TRANSLATING ANIMAL STUDIES TO HUMAN DISEASE

Clinical trials are unequivocally the ultimate translational tool despite being a challenge to design, fund, and conduct. Nonetheless, animal experiments have proven indispensable in the study of human diseases. In the scope of this article, the use of rat models in the study of human stroke treatment research represents a powerful translational variable. Rodent models permit manipulation of various variables while extending control over environmental factors, all of which have greatly advanced our mechanistic understanding of ischemic stroke pathophysiology.

Despite this progress, gaps exist in translating animal findings to the clinic with respect to applicable therapies.

In the context of exercise-onset dependent recovery from ischemic stroke, timing is proven to be a conundrum that limits our interpretation of the vast animal studies to humans. Morc specifically, the precise correlation of ischemic time between human and rodents remains unknown. However, it is clear that the tolerable duration of primate and human brain ischemia is considerably longer (6-8 h) than of rats [38]. Secondly, consider that current laboratory studies utilizing rat models are often implementing post-ischemic early exercise between 24-48 hours [39-43]. There is no doubt that the implementation of exercise at 24 hours in ischemic injured rats may not be early enough to simulate human conditions, considering the significantly shorter life span of a rat. This also implicates that the critical period, time course in which the ischemic brain is most sensitive to the beneficial effects of exercise, in animal stroke studies may be different from the critical period in human stroke. Consequently, the age of the animal was found to be a key factor in discerning the neuroplasticity related molecular profile and onset of its expression, which may be an important factor to consider in the translation of these findings to humans.

Current Debate on the Optimal Use of Exercise

How Early Is Early Exercise

Several factors impact the healing capacity of exercise as related to brain injury. Among them include onset of exercise which can have profound effects on prognosis of surviving stroke patients.

As alluded to previously, many guidelines pertaining to physical therapy and rehabilitation for stroke patients recommend early physical activity and ambulation at the least. As indicated above, clinical studies are applying therapy to patients as early as 18hrs post stroke [29, 30, 44, 45].

Concomitantly, researchers have employed animal models such as the middle cerebral artery occlusion (MCAO) rat models to assist in the delineation of the earliest time frame in which exercise therapy is beneficial rather than detrimental. The earliest documented exercise treatment for MCAO ischemic rat models is 24h [42, 46, 47]. Exercises employed include repetitive and motor skill training [42, 46, 48]. Some studies exposed animals to enriched environments constituting various physical activities [46] as well as force animals to use their impaired limb immediately following surgery [49, 50]. One study defined early training from 0-6 days [51]. Studying the therapeutic impact of various onsets of physical activity/exercise on stroke outcome is key to delineating the window of opportunity in which to reap the optimal benefits of exercise-mediated therapeutic intervention post-stroke. Needless to say, this can have profound effect on contemporary exercise-mediated treatment for patients suffering from various brain injury.

Early Exercise May Be Good or Bad

The rising interest in the potential therapeutic implications of exercise-mediated functional recovery in stroke patients has sparked the pursuit of defining the necessary time frame in which to optimize the benefits of exercise. The plethora of studies that have populated this discipline have led to conclusions short of unanimity. Although several studies have substantiated the beneficial effects of early exercise on recovery from cerebral ischemia [52-57] or hemorrhage [58] in animal models, there are some that contradict those findings by suggesting that early training exacerbates brain damage post stroke [9-11]. This section seeks to navigate through some of these studies.

Animal models are an invaluable tool used to simulate various human brain injuries. The MCAO induced ischemic rat model is one such model onto which the stroke outcome of various early training regimens is immensely investigated. In one study, animals that were administered treadmill training 24h post-surgery for one week exhibited reduced infarct volume and improved neurological function. Early treadmill training may mediate recovery of motor function by re-establishing the normal motor patterns during the sensitive period soon after brain injury [42]. Similar results were observed in the intracerebral hemorrhage (ICH) animal model that underwent early exercise training beginning 24h. These animals exhibited enhanced neurological recovery void of increases in hematoma expansion and edema volume unlike animals that underwent exercise after 1 week [59]. Consistently, forced early exercise on a running wheel led to improvements in functional outcome after focal cortical lesions with no change in lesion volume [60].

Likewise, when placed in an enriched environment 24h post-surgery, MCAO induced ischemic rats showed improved functional outcome without sustaining changes in infarct volume [46, 47].

Additionally, early exercise is shown to promote recovery from ischemic stroke in an intensity-dependent manner [61] with mild to moderate intensity proving beneficial and severe exercise intensity proving to be detrimental [62]. It is thought that a milder training intensity, as in treadmill training for 30 min per day [42], promotes reorganization of relevant cortical representation areas leading to motor functional improvements [63].

The aforementioned outcomes support early exercise as therapeutic to recovery from ischemic brain injury in an intensity dependent manner.

Early exercise following cerebral ischemia may not be entirely ameliorating. Some studies have labeled a period immediately after brain injury (0-6 days) as the early phase.

The early phase was identified as a vulnerable period; henceforth, early physical activity implemented here produced a negative outcome in functional recovery, lesion volume, and lesion-induced up-regulation of plasticity-related proteins [49, 64-66]. Additionally, a number of studies have demonstrated use-dependent exacerbation of brain damage in animals with unilateral lesion to the forelimb representation area of the sensorimotor cortex. In one such study, the unaffected limbs of such rats were immediately immobilized for 14 days following cerebral damage to force the overuse of the affected limb. These animals exhibited the largest behavioral deficits and the longest recovery period compared to when the impaired limb was immobilized. Meanwhile, the latter condition displayed only slightly larger and longer-lasting behavioral deficits [50]. In addition to slowing functional recovery, forced overuse of the impaired forelimb for 7 days resulted in expansion of the lesion and compromised functional recovery [49]. Even without forced use of the impaired limb, simply exposure of MCAO induced ischemic rats to an enriched environment and administration specific training 24h post-surgery was sufficient to exacerbate cortical tissue loss [64] thus suggesting that perhaps early training may indeed exacerbate brain damage [49, 50, 64].

Nonetheless, these studies stress the onset-dependent role of early exercise in stroke outcome, henceforth, placing importance on deciphering the confines of the window in which physical activity is beneficial rather than detrimental to ischemic tissue and subsequent functional recovery and rehabilitation.

Late Exercise in Rat Models

As in the case of early exercise mediated therapy, effects of late exercise therapy on various brain injury animal models pose similar extent of diverse outcomes. Take for instance the study that administered treadmill training to animals one week after MCAO-induced ischemia; no significant changes in infarct volume or neurological function was noted when compared to spontaneous recovery [42].

Additionally, when animals were forced to overuse their afflicted limb a week after lesion to the representative sensorimotor cortex, impaired recovery ensued although without any change in lesion volume [49].

On the other hand, delayed voluntary exercise following TBI (14-20 days) was characterized by up-regulated BDNF and improved cognitive function [51]. Up-regulation was also evident in downstream effectors of BDNF in both the dorsal hippocampus and cerebral cortex [51, 67-69].

MOLECULAR AND PHYSIOLOGICAL BASIS OF EARLY EXERCISE-MEDIATED RECOVERY

Neuroprotective Capacity of Early Exercise and Its Potential Role in Rehabilitative Functional Recovery

To understand how early exercise can potentially mediate or hinder recovery at the molecular and physiological level, a brief description of the ischemic cascade characteristic of stroke as well as TBI is warranted. Despite the difference in their initial insults, TBI and stroke share similar mechanisms that underline their pathophysiology such as excitotoxicity, oxidative stress, ROS, apoptosis, and inflammation [70]. Henceforth, TBI studies have been invaluable to advancing our understanding of effects of early exercise on stroke outcome and vice versa. The ischemic cascade ignited by stroke onset, a process similar to TBI, is a highly complex mechanism. Depending on the severity of the ischemia, brain cells may respond differently. However, despite this variation, there is a general process that all vulnerable brain cells undergo.

Recall that neurons in the ischemic core undergo apoptosis; however, it is the vulnerable neurons/tissue of the peri-ischemic core area (the penumbra) that undergo the aforementioned reversible debilitating energy consuming metabolic alternations. In agreement, this region is marked by elevated glucose metabolism that can last up to 6 h upon reperfusion [71].

Henceforth, the vulnerable penumbra can be potentially rescued through neuroprotective therapies which is the basis for rehabilitation.

Currently, a clinically effective neuroprotectant is yet to be uncovered, although exercise-mediated recovery is a frequent recourse. The rehabilitative capacity of exercise training on stroke patients is widely recognized and is applied in many physical therapy programs today. As previously eluded to, many such guidelines recommend early physical/exercise therapy. However, as seen in the previous section, the parameters under which early rehabilitative exercise is deemed maximally neuroprotective and functionally beneficial to stroke patients is yet to be characterized. This section seeks to briefly describe the ischemic cascade characteristic of stroke and the potential influence of early exercise on the cascade.

Metabolic disorder. From a metabolic point of view, the immediate repercussions of oxygen deprivation incurred in acute stroke is impaired aerobic mitochondrial oxidative phosphorylation of glucose, the primary energy source for neuronal activity.

Hereafter, surviving brain cells respond by increasing anaerobic glycolysis (hyper-glycolysis), a pathway involved in the initial catabolism of glucose [72, 73]. Hyper-glycolysis is reflected in elevated levels of its key enzymes [74] such as phosphofructo-kinase (PFK), lactate dehydrogenase (LDH), and phosphorylated adenosine monophosphate kinase (pAMPK) as well as up-regulation of glucose uptake transporters 1 and 3 (GLUT1 and 3) [75]. Hyper-glycolysis also contributes to metabolic acidosis via lactate accumulation, a by-product of anaerobic glycolysis [76]. Meanwhile, the mitochondria reacts to this hypoxic crisis by increasing the activity of the rate-limiting electron transport chain (ETC) enzyme cytochrome c oxidase (CcO). Consequently, the mitochondrial membrane potential is hyperpolarized to levels that support non-physiological ROS production upon reperfusion [77]. ROS production has shown to cause cellular damage and death in cerebral ischemia and reperfusion [77]. Henceforth, conditions that support ROS production is not a cultivating environment for vulnerable brain cells [11]. Adding to the metabolic disarray, brain cells exhibit uncontrolled energy consuming activity of ion pumps. This facilitates a change in membrane potential supporting liberation of excitatory neurotransmitters such as glutamate [73, 78]. In essence, ischemia brought about by various brain injuries including stroke, is characterized by altered metabolism wherein energy supply is compromised despite an increased demand for it. This creates energy imbalance apt for oxidative stress leading to neural damage and loss-of-function [11].

Metabolic response to early exercise. It is thought that perhaps conditions that exacerbate the hyper-metabolic milieu characterized in the early ischemic period of stroke, such as physical activity and exercise, may have negative effects on the vulnerable penumbra. Consider that PFK-1, a key AMP-activated glycolytic enzyme isoform found in neurons and astrocytes [79], is increased in response to exercise. Likewise, the active form of AMPK was also found to be increased following exercise thus indicating that exercise drives catabolism to meet elevated energy demands [73]. Furthermore, subjecting animals to exercise training [80] or simply exposing them to enriched environments [81] was sufficient to induce angiogenesis, thus exemplifying the body's need to meet increased energy demands. Clinical studies have also established a significant increase in energy demand to sustain the hemiparetic gait of stroke patients [23, 24]. Henceforth, animals forced to use their impaired limb during the early ischemic period, which is marked by hyperactivity in the already vulnerable penumbra, may further tip the energy balance toward a state of deficiency. This sets the stage for transient episodes of hypoxia and reserved recovery [82-84].

The associated metabolic and neurochemical alterations following injury hinders exercise-induced neuroplasticity-associated molecular changes [51]. Eluding to this, cortical stimulation post-TBI elicits a metabolic response that may further increase cortical degeneration [85]. This finding posits that the brain may be undergoing metabolic changes during the first week post-injury, which can strongly affect the outcome of exercise-mediated therapies [86-88].

Henceforth, immature onset of exercise can divert energy stores inappropriately from the much needed production of synaptic plasticity-related molecules to meet metabolic demands of exercise on an already energetically compromised brain. Exercise increases energy demands (primarily in the hippocampus, motor cortex, and striatum) [89], regional cerebral blood flow [90, 91], and extracellular lactate [92].

BDNF signaling pathways. The resulting energy imbalance facilitates the activation of various brain cell death pathways as well as regenerative efforts following stroke. Neurotrophic factors play a key role as neuroprotectants after cerebral insult. Among them include nerve growth factor (NGF) and brain-derived nerve growth factor (BDNF) both of which promote cell growth and enhance neuronal activity [93, 94]. Although a growth factor, midkine has neurotrophic properties implicated in repair of several tissues and found to be expressed in the early stages of cerebral infarction [95].

The BDNF signaling pathway is thought to be a key mediator of angiogenesis [96], neurogenesis [97, 98], and synaptic plasticity [99] all the while serving as a neuroprotective agent [100, 101]. Additionally, this pathway is known for inhibiting the pathological processes of neurotoxicity, apoptosis, and inflammation [102]. In other words, BDNF plays a critical role in post-stroke recovery. Despite this, the effects of stroke on BDNF production has not been completely delineated. Studies indicate an increase in BDNF production at the infarct and peri-infarct sites at least a week following stroke [103, 104]. Aside from neurons, BDNF is also produced by non-neuronal cells such as endothelial cells of microvessels, microglial cells, and astrocytes in the ischemic brain. Additionally, BDNF production by these non-neural cells is positively correlated with infarct size [105].

The signaling pathway involving BDNF is quite diverse. Mature BDNF is cleaved from proBDNF by tissue-type plasminogen activator (tPA). This change allows BDNF to bind to the TrkB receptor enabling the activation of many intracellular signaling pathways including the Ras/extracellular signal regulated protein kinase (ERK), the phophatidylionsitol-3-OH (PI3K)/AKT kinase, and the Ca^{2+} activated kinase (CaMKII) pathways [106]. These pathways converge to manipulate CREB production, phosphorylation, and function [107] which in turn affects transcription of cell survival genes. The AKT pathway indirectly manipulates CREB by deactivating its antagonist transcription factor FOXO3 known to induce transcription of apoptotic proteins [108], henceforth indirectly promoting cell survival [109] (Figure 2).

Another downstream effector of the BDNF-TrkB signaling pathways is synapsin I, a synaptic trafficking protein expressed in axon terminals, involved in the facilitation of neurotransmitter release, axonal growth, and the maintenance of synaptic connection [110, 111]. Its synthesis and phosphorylation is affected by CaMKII and ERK signaling (Figure 2). ICH studies have indicated that the BDNF-TrkB signaling pathway is activated in the peri-hemorrhagic area. Significant increases were observed on day 7 which subsided close to normal levels by day 14. This suggests that the BDNF-TrkB signaling pathway may be involved in the brain repair process, although levels present maybe insufficient for complete functional recovery [112].

BDNF-induced neuroplasticity. Exercise is neuroprotective and can induce neuroplasticity in many CNS disorders including stroke [113, 114]. It is linked to slowing cognitive decay [115], neuronal protection against ischemia [53], enhanced neurogenesis [116], and improved learning capabilities [116, 117] making exercise a viable candidate for improving prognosis in ischemic brain injury [118]. The benefits incurred through exercise are strongly linked to increases in neurotropic factors such as BDNF [56]. Increases are seen throughout the brain, especially in the hippocampus and posterior cortex [119]. It is thought that persistent BDNF expression is crucial for recovery from ischemic/hemorrhagic stroke, the expression of which can be prolonged through exercise. In fact, exercises such as treadmill training have shown enhanced and prolonged activated BNDF-TrkB pathway in the peri-hemorrhagic areas of ICH-induced rats, suggesting the important role of rehabilitation by treadmill exercise [112]. Increases in BDNF are attributed to enhancement of functional recovery in MCAO animals exposed to enriched environment and exercise [120]. Consistently, voluntary wheel running exercise increased downstream effectors of BDNF such as PI3K, PKB/AKT, CREB, and TrkB in the hippocampus [121].

Exercise has also shown to increase the activity of tPA which is responsible for the conversion of proBDNF to mBDNF. This became evident when inhibited tPA activity reduced exercise-induced effects of BDNF. Subsequently inhibition of TrkB receptor and its downstream signaling effectors ERK, Akt, and CaMKII followed. Furthermore, exercise-induced expression of plasticity markers synapsin I and growth-associated protein 43 (GAP-43) were also reversed.

This finding implicates the hippocampal plasticity effects of exercise to BDNF processing and henceforth, TrkB signalling [106].

It is well known that endogenous BDNF and its downstream effectors are up-regulated and functional recovery enhanced post-TBI when running wheel exercise was delayed for 14 days. However, when exercise was administered sooner (0-6 days) post-TBI, endogenous BDNF levels were reduced and associated cognitive impairment were observed. All the while, sham animals exhibited hippocampal BDNF upregulation proportional to the amount of exercise [51]. In addition to reduced BDNF expression, pCREB expression was also reduced and associated impaired learning ensued with early voluntary exercise (0-6 days) [65]. It is possible that the stress of increased metabolic demand imposed by exercise may have adverse effects early after brain injury by further injuring the already compromised tissue.

According to amassing literature, exercise-induced changes in gene expression are perpetuated via modulation of the BDNF system, promoting cell survival and inhibiting apoptosis as discussed previously. Other interactions that converge onto this pathway include the Ca^{2+} activated kinase, CaMKII, which is observed to be up-regulated during acute exercise [122]. Additional up-regulated genes in rats that underwent voluntary running exercise include those involved in synaptic trafficking (syntaxin, synapsin I, and synaptotagmin), neurotransmitter systems, and other signal transduction pathways [122]. Exercise-induced BDNF-TrkB interaction also activates the MAP-K cascade which leads to downstream phosphorylation of CREB [123] and protein synapsin I [124-126] Among its many roles, CREB induces transcription of target genes, including BDNK [123] related to long-term plasticity [127] and memory [128].

Exercise and Neuroplasticity: Synaptogenesis, Neurogenesis, and Angiogenesis

As eluded to in previous sections, exercise promotes changes in the brain at a neuroanatomical level. Evidence from both human and animal studies converge to suggest that physical exercise promotes neuroplasticity in certain areas of the brain [129]. In the context of ischemic stroke, recovery of motor function involves relearning of motor skills which is a neuroplasticity-mediated process [130]. This recovery process can occur spontaneously post-stroke but can also be enhanced with appropriate rehabilitation [63, 131, 132].

This section will explore the response to post-ischemic stroke with respect to neuroplasticity and the potential role of exercise as a facilitator.

Neurogenesis. Animal studies have established that voluntary aerobic exercise can induce formation of new neurons within the hippocampus of adult mice concomitant to enhanced learning.

This process, occurring primarily in the subventricular zone (SVZ) and subgranular zone (SGZ) of the hippocampus of the adult brain [133, 134], is hampered in the elderly who are a highly susceptible to stroke [135-138].

In addition to its preventative capacity, exercise can also reverse deleterious consequences of aging [134, 139]. Like exercise, environment enrichment, growth factors, and even pathological process such as ischemic stroke can induce neurogenesis. Experimental stroke in animal studies have shown newborn neuron migration into ischemic brain regions. Similarly, stroke patients have expressed markers associated with newborn neurons in the ischemic penumbra preferentially near the vicinity of blood vessels [140].

As discussed previously, trophic factors are key players in adult neurogenesis. In addition to BDNF, notable trophic factors include basic fibroblast growth factor (bFGF-2), epidermal growth factor (EGF), insulin like growth factor I (IGF-I), and vascular endothelial growth factor (VEGF). For instance, intraverebroventricular administration of BDNF increased neurogenesis in the adult olfactory bulb [141] and striatum [142].

In agreement, BDNF knockout mice failed to show enhanced neurogenesis following environmental enrichment [143]. As seen with the BDNF signaling pathway, exercise is also associated with increased genes expression of FGF [68, 144] and NGF in the hippocampus [145].

Angiogenesis. Angiogenesis and neurogenesis are closely associated processes [146-149]. For instance, it has been demonstrated that new cells of the dentate gyrus associate with blood vessels [146] and respond to vascular growth factors such as VEGF [150, 151]. Additionally, increased adult neurogenesis [152] and a reversal of aging-associated decrease in neurogenesis [153] was observed with peripheral infusion of IGF-1 [145].

Like neurogenesis, angiogenesis can also be induced in the CNS by hypoxia and ischemia seen in stroke [154]. It is well established that physical exercise increases angiogenesis throughout the brain [155-158] which is proposed to be mediated by IGF and VEGF. Running exercises enhance IGF gene expression [159, 160], increase serum IGF [161] and VEGF [162].

Consistently, inhibition of VEGF and IGF-1 failed to show enhanced neurogenesis observed with running [145, 162, 163].

Synaptogenesis. The penumbra is the site of active structural and functional remodeling. It is characterized by factors that induce axonal sprouting [132, 164, 165] and support elaboration of dendrites and spines [166, 167]. Positive factors involved in this rewiring process include: glialderived synaptogenic thrombospondin 1 and 2 [168] and growth-related proteins such as GAP43, mArCKS, CAP23 and growth factors [169-171]. This process is regulated by factors that inhibit outgrowths such as extracellular matrix factors NOGO [172-174], chondroitin sulphate proteoglycan 64, ephrin A5, semaphorin 3A and neuropilin 1, and EPH receptors and ligands [175]. Interestingly, expression of these factors are temporally related such that growth stimulatory factors precede inhibitory factors after stroke [175].

Window of opportunity for neural plasticity in the post-ischemic brain. As eluded to previously, neuroplasticity can occur spontaneously following an injury as seen when the corresponding cortical area of a transected median nerve of adult owls or squirrel monkeys was completely occupied by new and expanded representations of surrounding skin fields [131].

Such cortical reorganization is no exception following stroke. For instance, adult mice in which focal ischemic stroke was induced in the forelimb sensorimotor cortex showed a re-emergence of forelimb-evoked depolarization from surrounding peri-infarct motor/hindlimb area as well as from the distant posteromedial retrosplenial cortex [132].

The existence of a critical period during which the brain is sensitive to exercise rehabilitation is a recurrent theme throughout this article. This concept was eluded to in the previous section pertaining to onset-dependent effects of exercise in animal models. Recall that proteins regarded as positive factors for neuroplasticity such glial-derived synaptogenic thrombospondin ½ [168] and proteins that promote synaptogenesis such GAP43 [170], CAP23 and mArCKS were highly expressed post-stroke. Meanwhile, Nogo-A [172], MAG, semaphoring 3A, CSPG [176], and neurocan [177] are thought to be factors that inhibit axonal outgrowth and sprouting. Taken conjunctively, it is hypothesized that an interplay between positive and negative factors that either promote or discourage neuroplasticity, respectively, might be an important determinant of this critical period.

Conclusion

Exercise-mediated rehabilitation therapy is unequivocally beneficial in the recovery of stroke survivors. However, the benefits incurred are variable in the scope of early exercise-mediated therapy. Animal studies utilizing various stroke models, particularly the MCAO rodent model, have investigated this phenomenon in functional recovery and have concluded that benefits can range from significant to detrimental. These findings have fueled the proposition of underlying time-dependent factors that that may negatively affect the beneficial outcomes of exercise following stroke. Animal studies have focused on deciphering the underlying mechanisms. Molecular perspective under study include the influences of the changing metabolic milieu following stroke, termed as metabolic disorder, and the dynamic signaling pathways involved in neuroplasticity, the cornerstone of functional recovery. Understanding the time-dependent interplay between these processes can perhaps provide a clue to the nature of the onset-dependent benefits of exercise and therefore advance the field of exercise rehabilitative therapy.

REFERENCES

[1] Lo, E. H., Dalkara, T., Moskowitz, M. A. Mechanisms, challenges and opportunities in stroke. *Nat. Rev. Neurosci.* 2003;4(5):399-415.

[2] Organization, W. H. *The top 10 causes of death 2014 [cited 2014 June 9].* Available from: http://www.who.int/mediacentre/factsheets/fs310/en/.

[3] Bamford, J., Dennis, M., Sandercock, P., Burn, J., Warlow, C. The frequency, causes and timing of death within 30 days of a first stroke: the Oxfordshire Community Stroke Project. *Journal of neurology, neurosurgery, and psychiatry.* 1990;53(10):824-9.

[4] Thrift, A. G., Dewey, H. M., Macdonell, R. A., McNeil, J. J., Donnan, G. A. Stroke incidence on the east coast of Australia: the North East Melbourne Stroke Incidence Study (NEMESIS). *Stroke; a journal of cerebral circulation.* 2000;31(9):2087-92.

[5] Almeida, O. P., Khan, K. M., Hankey, G. J., Yeap, B. B., Golledge, J., Flicker, L. 150 minutes of vigorous physical activity per week predicts survival and successful ageing: a population-based 11-year longitudinal study of 12 201 older Australian men. *British journal of sports medicine.* 2014;48(3):220-5.

[6] Mizutani, K., Sonoda, S., Yamada, K., Beppu, H., Shimpo, K. Alteration of protein expression profile following voluntary exercise in the perilesional cortex of rats with focal cerebral infarction. *Brain research.* 2011;1416:61-8.

[7] Arya, K. N., Pandian, S., Verma, R., Garg, R. K. Movement therapy induced neural reorganization and motor recovery in stroke: a review. *Journal of bodywork and movement therapies*. 2011;15(4):528-37.

[8] Johansson, B. B. Brain plasticity and stroke rehabilitation. The Willis lecture. *Stroke; a journal of cerebral circulation*. 2000;31(1):223-30.

[9] Astrup, J., Siesjo, B. K., Symon, L. Thresholds in cerebral ischemia - the ischemic penumbra. *Stroke; a journal of cerebral circulation*. 1981; 12 (6):723-5.

[10] Allen, C. L., Bayraktutan, U. Oxidative stress and its role in the pathogenesis of ischaemic stroke. *International journal of stroke: official journal of the International Stroke Society*. 2009;4(6):461-70.

[11] Siesjo, B. K., Katsura, K. I., Kristian, T., Li, P. A., Siesjo, P. Molecular mechanisms of acidosis-mediated damage. *Acta neurochirurgica Supplement*. 1996;66:8-14.

[12] Pang, M. Y., Eng, J. J., Dawson, A. S., Gylfadottir, S. The use of aerobic exercise training in improving aerobic capacity in individuals with stroke: a meta-analysis. *Clinical rehabilitation*. 2006;20(2):97-111.

[13] Stewart, K. C., Cauraugh, J. H., Summers, J. J. Bilateral movement training and stroke rehabilitation: a systematic review and meta-analysis. *Journal of the neurological sciences*. 2006;244(1-2):89-95.

[14] Daly, J. J., Ruff, R. L. Construction of efficacious gait and upper limb functional interventions based on brain plasticity evidence and model-based measures for stroke patients. *The Scientific World Journal*. 2007; 7:2031-45.

[15] Jauch, E. C., Cucchiara, B., Adeoye, O., Meurer, W., Brice, J., Chan, Y. Y., et al. Part 11: adult stroke: 2010 American Heart Association Guidelines for Cardiopulmonary Resuscitation and Emergency Cardiovascular Care. *Circulation*. 2010;122(18 Suppl. 3):S818-28.

[16] Duncan, P. W., Zorowitz, R., Bates, B., Choi, J. Y., Glasberg, J. J., Graham, G. D., et al. Management of Adult Stroke Rehabilitation Care: a clinical practice guideline. *Stroke; a journal of cerebral circulation*. 2005;36(9):e100-43.

[17] Fisher, S. V., Gullickson, G., Jr. Energy cost of ambulation in health and disability: a literature review. *Archives of physical medicine and rehabilitation*. 1978;59(3):124-33.

[18] Nijland, R., van Wegen, E., van der Krogt, H., Bakker, C., Buma, F., Klomp, A., et al. Characterizing the protocol for early modified constraint-induced movement therapy in the EXPLICIT-stroke trial.

Physiotherapy research international: the journal for researchers and clinicians in physical therapy. 2013;18(1):1-15.

[19] Mol, V. J., Baker, C. A. Activity intolerance in the geriatric stroke patient. *Rehabilitation nursing: the official journal of the Association of Rehabilitation Nurses*. 1991;16(6):337-43.

[20] Potempa, K., Braun, L. T., Tinknell, T., Popovich, J. Benefits of aerobic exercise after stroke. *Sports medicine* (Auckland, NZ). 1996;21(5):337-46.

[21] Macko, R. F., Smith, G. V., Dobrovolny, C. L., Sorkin, J. D., Goldberg, A. P., Silver, K. H. Treadmill training improves fitness reserve in chronic stroke patients. *Archives of physical medicine and rehabilitation*. 2001;82(7):879-84.

[22] Meek, C., Pollock, A., Potter, J., Langhorne, P. A systematic review of exercise trials post stroke. *Clinical rehabilitation*. 2003;17(1):6-13.

[23] Corcoran, P. J., Jebsen, R. H., Brengelmann, G. L., Simons, B. C. Effects of plastic and metal leg braces on speed and energy cost of hemiparetic ambulation. *Archives of physical medicine and rehabilitation*. 1970;51(2):69-77.

[24] Gersten, J. W., Orr, W. External work of walking in hemiparetic patients. *Scandinavian journal of rehabilitation medicine*. 1971;3(1):85-8.

[25] Olney, S. J., Monga, T. N., Costigan, P. A. Mechanical energy of walking of stroke patients. *Archives of physical medicine and rehabilitation*. 1986;67(2):92-8.

[26] Ivey, F. M., Hafer-Macko, C. E., Macko, R. F. Exercise rehabilitation after stroke. *NeuroRx: the journal of the American Society for Experimental NeuroTherapeutics*. 2006;3(4):439-50.

[27] Van Peppen, R. P., Kwakkel, G., Wood-Dauphinee, S., Hendriks, H. J., Van der Wees, P. J., Dekker, J. The impact of physical therapy on functional outcomes after stroke: what's the evidence? *Clinical rehabilitation*. 2004;18(8):833-62.

[28] Ada, L., Dorsch, S., Canning, C. G. Strengthening interventions increase strength and improve activity after stroke: a systematic review. *The Australian journal of physiotherapy*. 2006;52(4):241-8.

[29] van Wijk, R., Cumming, T., Churilov, L., Donnan, G., Bernhardt, J. An early mobilization protocol successfully delivers more and earlier therapy to acute stroke patients: further results from phase II of AVERT. *Neurorehabilitation and neural repair*. 2012;26(1):20-6.

[30] Cumming, T. B., Thrift, A. G., Collier, J. M., Churilov, L., Dewey, H. M., Donnan, G. A., et al. Very early mobilization after stroke fast-tracks return to walking: further results from the phase II AVERT randomized controlled trial. *Stroke; a journal of cerebral circulation*. 2011;42(1): 153-8.

[31] Langhorne, P., Stott, D., Knight, A., Bernhardt, J., Barer, D., Watkins, C. Very early rehabilitation or intensive telemetry after stroke: a pilot randomised trial. *Cerebrovascular diseases* (Basel, Switzerland). 2010; 29(4):352-60.

[32] Maulden, S. A., Gassaway, J., Horn, S. D., Smout, R. J., DeJong, G. Timing of initiation of rehabilitation after stroke. *Archives of physical medicine and rehabilitation*. 2005;86(12 Suppl. 2):S34-s40.

[33] Di Lauro, A., Pellegrino, L., Savastano, G., Ferraro, C., Fusco, M., Balzarano, F., et al. A randomized trial on the efficacy of intensive rehabilitation in the acute phase of ischemic stroke. *Journal of neurology*. 2003;250(10):1206-8.

[34] Adams, H. P., Jr., Adams, R. J., Brott, T., del Zoppo, G. J., Furlan, A., Goldstein, L. B., et al. Guidelines for the early management of patients with ischemic stroke: A scientific statement from the Stroke Council of the American Stroke Association. *Stroke; a journal of cerebral circulation*. 2003;34(4):1056-83.

[35] Bernhardt, J., Indredavik, B., Dewey, H., Langhorne, P., Lindley, R., Donnan, G., et al. Mobilisation 'in bed' is not mobilisation. *Cerebrovascular diseases* (Basel, Switzerland). 2007;24(1):157-8; author reply 9.

[36] Diserens, K., Michel, P., Bogousslavsky, J. Early mobilisation after stroke: Review of the literature. *Cerebrovascular diseases* (Basel, Switzerland). 2006;22(2-3):183-90.

[37] Byl, N. N., Pitsch, E. A., Abrams, G. M. Functional outcomes can vary by dose: learning-based sensorimotor training for patients stable poststroke. *Neurorehabilitation and neural repair*. 2008;22(5):494-504.

[38] Zivin, J. A. Factors determining the therapeutic window for stroke. *Neurology*. 1998;50(3):599-603.

[39] Jiang, X. F., Zhang, T., Sy, C., Nie, B. B., Hu, X. Y., Ding, Y. Dynamic metabolic changes after permanent cerebral ischemia in rats with/ without post-stroke exercise: a positron emission tomography (PET) study. *Neurological research*. 2014;36(5):475-82.

[40] Yang, Y. R., Chang, H. C., Wang, P. S., Wang, R. Y. Motor performance improved by exercises in cerebral ischemic rats. *Journal of motor behavior*. 2012;44(2):97-103.

[41] Liu, N., Huang, H., Lin, F., Chen, A., Zhang, Y., Chen, R., et al. Effects of treadmill exercise on the expression of netrin-1 and its receptors in rat brain after cerebral ischemia. *Neuroscience*. 2011;194:349-58.

[42] Yang, Y. R., Wang, R. Y., Wang, P. S. Early and late treadmill training after focal brain ischemia in rats. *Neurosci. Lett*. 2003;339(2):91-4.

[43] Choe, M. A., An, G. J., Lee, Y. K., Im, J. H., Choi-Kwon, S., Heitkemper, M. Effect of early low-intensity exercise on rat hind-limb muscles following acute ischemic stroke. *Biol. Res. Nurs*. 2006;7(3): 163-74.

[44] Bernhardt, J., Dewey, H., Thrift, A., Collier, J., Donnan, G. A very early rehabilitation trial for stroke (AVERT): phase II safety and feasibility. *Stroke; a journal of cerebral circulation*. 2008;39(2):390-6.

[45] Craig, L. E., Bernhardt, J., Langhorne, P., Wu, O. Early mobilization after stroke: an example of an individual patient data meta-analysis of a complex intervention. *Stroke; a journal of cerebral circulation*. 2010;41 (11):2632-6.

[46] Johansson, B. B., Ohlsson, A. L. Environment, social interaction, and physical activity as determinants of functional outcome after cerebral infarction in the rat. *Experimental neurology*. 1996;139(2):322-7.

[47] Ohlsson, A. L., Johansson, B. B. Environment influences functional outcome of cerebral infarction in rats. *Stroke; a journal of cerebral circulation*. 1995;26(4):644-9.

[48] Tamakoshi, K., Ishida, A., Takamatsu, Y., Hamakawa, M., Nakashima, H., Shimada, H., et al. Motor skills training promotes motor functional recovery and induces synaptogenesis in the motor cortex and striatum after intracerebral hemorrhage in rats. *Behavioural brain research*. 2014; 260:34-43.

[49] Humm, J. L., Kozlowski, D. A., James, D. C., Gotts, J. E., Schallert, T. Use-dependent exacerbation of brain damage occurs during an early post-lesion vulnerable period. *Brain Res*. 1998;783:286-92.

[50] Kozlowski, D. A. J. D., Schallert, T. Use-dependent exaggeration of neuronal injury after unilateral sensorimotor cortex lesions. *J. Neurosci*. 1996;16(15):4776-86.

[51] Griesbach, G. S., Hovda, D. A., Molteni, R., Wu, A., Gomez-Pinilla, F. Voluntary exercise following traumatic brain injury: brain-derived

neurotrophic factor upregulation and recovery of function. *Neuroscience*. 2004;125(1):129-39.

[52] Matsuda, F., Sakakima, H., Yoshida, Y. The effects of early exercise on brain damage and recovery after focal cerebral infarction in rats. *Acta Physiologica*. 2011;201(2):275-87.

[53] Stummer, W., Weber, K., Tranmer, B., Baethmann, A., Kempski, O. Reduced mortality and brain damage after locomotor activity in gerbil forebrain ischemia. *Stroke; a journal of cerebral circulation*. 1994;25 (9):1862-9.

[54] Stummer, W., Baethmann, A., Murr, R., Schurer, L., Kempski, O. S. Cerebral protection against ischemia by locomotor activity in gerbils. Underlying mechanisms. *Stroke; a journal of cerebral circulation*. 1995; 26(8):1423-9; discussion 30.

[55] Wang, R. Y., Yang, Y. R., Yu, S. M. Protective effects of treadmill training on infarction in rats. *Brain research*. 2001;922(1):140-3.

[56] Ang, E. T., Wong, P. T. H., Moochhala, S., Ng, Y. K. Neuroprotection associated with running: Is it a result of increased endogenous neurotrophic factors? *Neuroscience*. 2003;118(2):335-45.

[57] Endres, M., Gertz, K., Lindauer, U., Katchanov, J., Schultze, J., Schrock, H., et al. Mechanisms of stroke protection by physical activity. *Ann. Neurol.* 2003;54(5):582-90.

[58] Park, J. W., Bang, M. S., Kwon, B. S., Park, Y. K., Kim, D. W., Shon, S. M., et al. Early treadmill training promotes motor function after hemorrhagic stroke in rats. *Neurosci. Lett.* 2010;471(2):104-8.

[59] Jang, D. P., Lee, S. H., Lee, S. Y., Park, C. W., Cho, Z. H., Kim, Y. B. Neural responses of rats in the forced swimming test: [F-18]FDG micro PET study. *Behavioural brain research*. 2009;203(1):43-7.

[60] Hart, C. L. D. G., Barth, T. M. Forced activity facilitates recovery of function following cortical lesions in rats. *Natl. Neurotr. Soc. Abstr.* 1997:101.

[61] Bland, S. T., Schallert, T., Strong, R., Aronowski, J., Grotta, J. C., Feeney, D. M. Early exclusive use of the affected forelimb after moderate transient focal ischemia in rats: functional and anatomic outcome. *Stroke; a journal of cerebral circulation*. 2000;31(5):1144-52.

[62] Lee, S. U., Kim, D. Y., Park, S. H., Choi, D. H., Park, H. W., Han, T. R. Mild to moderate early exercise promotes recovery from cerebral ischemia in rats. *The Canadian journal of neurological sciences Le journal canadien des sciences neurologiques*. 2009;36(4):443-9.

[63] Nudo, R. J., Wise, B. M., SiFuentes, F., Milliken, G. W. Neural substrates for the effects of rehabilitative training on motor recovery after ischemic infarct. *Science* (New York, NY). 1996;272(5269):1791-4.

[64] Risedal, A. Z. J., Johansson, B. B. Early training may exacerbate brain damage after focal brain ischemia in the rat. *J. Cereb. Blood Flow Metab.* 1999;19:997-1003.

[65] Griesbach, G. S., Gomez-Pinilla, F., Hovda, D. A. The upregulation of plasticity-related proteins following TBI is disrupted with acute voluntary exercise. *Brain research.* 2004;1016(2):154-62.

[66] Griesbach, G. S., Hovda, D. A., Molteni, R., Gomez-Pinilla, F. Alterations in BDNF and synapsin I within the occipital cortex and hippocampus after mild traumatic brain injury in the developing rat: reflections of injury-induced neuroplasticity. *Journal of neurotrauma.* 2002;19(7):803-14.

[67] Neeper, S. A., Gomez-Pinilla, F., Choi, J., Cotman, C. Exercise and brain neurotrophins. *Nature.* 1995;373(6510):109.

[68] Gomez-Pinilla, F., So, V., Kesslak, J. P. Spatial learning and physical activity contribute to the induction of fibroblast growth factor: neural substrates for increased cognition associated with exercise. *Neuroscience.* 1998;85(1):53-61.

[69] Gomez-Pinilla, F., So, V., Kesslak, J. P. Spatial learning induces neurotrophin receptor and synapsin I in the hippocampus. *Brain research.* 2001;904(1):13-9.

[70] Bramlett, H. M., Dietrich, W. D. Pathophysiology of cerebral ischemia and brain trauma[colon] Similarities and differences. *Journal of cerebral blood flow and metabolism: official journal of the International Society of Cerebral Blood Flow and Metabolism.* 2004;24(2):133-50.

[71] Chen, H., Song, Y. S., Chan, P. H. Inhibition of NADPH oxidase is neuroprotective after ischemia-reperfusion. *Journal of cerebral blood flow and metabolism: official journal of the International Society of Cerebral Blood Flow and Metabolism.* 2009;29(7):1262-72.

[72] Memezawa, H., Minamisawa, H., Smith, M. L., Siesjo, B. K. Ischemic penumbra in a model of reversible middle cerebral artery occlusion in the rat. *Experimental brain research.* 1992;89(1):67-78.

[73] Schurr, A. Energy metabolism, stress hormones and neural recovery from cerebral ischemia/hypoxia. *Neurochem. Int.* 2002;41(1):1-8.

[74] Carling, D. The AMP-activated protein kinase cascade - A unifying system for energy control. *Trends in Biochemical Sciences*. 2004;29(1): 18-24.

[75] Kinni, H., Guo, M., Ding, J. Y., Konakondla, S., Dornbos, D., 3rd, Tran, R., et al. Cerebral metabolism after forced or voluntary physical exercise. *Brain research.* 2011;1388:48-55.

[76] Gladden, L. B. Lactate metabolism: A new paradigm for the third millennium. *Journal of Physiology*. 2004;558(1):5-30.

[77] Chan, P. H. Reactive oxygen radicals in signaling and damage in the ischemic brain. *Journal of cerebral blood flow and metabolism: official journal of the International Society of Cerebral Blood Flow and Metabolism.* 2001;21(1):2-14.

[78] Floyd, R. A., Towner, R. A., He, T., Hensley, K., Maples, K. R. Translational research involving oxidative stress and diseases of aging. *Free radical biology and medicine*. 2011;51(5):931-41.

[79] Almeida, A., Moncada, S., Bolanos, J. P. Nitric oxide switches on glycolysis through the AMP protein kinase and 6-phosphofructo-2-kinase pathway. *Nature cell biology*. 2004;6(1):45-51.

[80] Black Jei, K. R., Anderson, B. J., Alcantara, A. A., Greenough, W. T. Learning causes synaptogenesis, whereas motor activity causes angiogenesis, in cerebellar cortex of adult rats. *Proc. Nati. Acad. Sci.* 1990;87:5568-72.

[81] Black, J. E., Zelazny, A. M., Greenough, W. T. Capillary and mitochondrial support of neural plasticity in adult rat visual cortex. *Experimental neurology*. 1991;111(2):204-9.

[82] Nedergaard, M., Hansen, A. J. Characterization of cortical depolarizations evoked in focal cerebral ischemia. *Journal of cerebral blood flow and metabolism: official journal of the International Society of Cerebral Blood Flow and Metabolism*. 1993;13(4):568-74.

[83] Back, T., Hoehn-Berlage, M., Kohno, K., Hossmann, K. A. Diffusion nuclear magnetic resonance imaging in experimental stroke. Correlation with cerebral metabolites. *Stroke; a journal of cerebral circulation*. 1994;25(2):494-500.

[84] Mies, G., Ishimaru, S., Xie, Y., Seo, K., Hossmann, K. A. Ischemic thresholds of cerebral protein synthesis and energy state following middle cerebral artery occlusion in rat. *Journal of cerebral blood flow and metabolism: official journal of the International Society of Cerebral Blood Flow and Metabolism.* 1991;11(5):753-61.

[85] Ip, E. Y., Zanier, E. R., Moore, A. H., Lee, S. M., Hovda, D. A. Metabolic, neurochemical, and histologic responses to vibrissa motor cortex stimulation after traumatic brain injury. *Journal of cerebral blood flow and metabolism: official journal of the International Society of Cerebral Blood Flow and Metabolism*. 2003;23(8):900-10.

[86] Fineman, I., Hovda, D. A., Smith, M., Yoshino, A., Becker, D. P. Concussive brain injury is associated with a prolonged accumulation of calcium: a 45Ca autoradiographic study. *Brain research*. 1993;624(1-2): 94-102.

[87] Ginsberg, M. D., Zhao, W., Alonso, O. F., Loor-Estades, J. Y., Dietrich, W. D., Busto, R. Uncoupling of local cerebral glucose metabolism and blood flow after acute fluid-percussion injury in rats. *The American journal of physiology*. 1997;272(6 Pt 2):H2859-68.

[88] Moore, A. H., Osteen, C. L., Chatziioannou, A. F., Hovda, D. A., Cherry, S. R. Quantitative assessment of longitudinal metabolic changes in vivo after traumatic brain injury in the adult rat using FDG-microPET. *Journal of cerebral blood flow and metabolism: official journal of the International Society of Cerebral Blood Flow and Metabolism*. 2000; 20 (10):1492-501.

[89] Vissing, J., Andersen, M., Diemer, N. H. Exercise-induced changes in local cerebral glucose utilization in the rat. *Journal of cerebral blood flow and metabolism: official journal of the International Society of Cerebral Blood Flow and Metabolism*. 1996;16(4):729-36.

[90] Gross, P. M., Marcus, M. L., Heistad, D. D. Regional distribution of cerebral blood flow during exercise in dogs. *Journal of applied physiology: respiratory, environmental and exercise physiology*. 1980; 48(2):213-7.

[91] Orgogozo, J. M., Larsen, B. Activation of the supplementary motor area during voluntary movement in man suggests it works as a supramotor area. *Science* (New York, NY). 1979;206(4420):847-50.

[92] De Bruin, L. A., Schasfoort, E. M., Steffens, A. B., Korf, J. Effects of stress and exercise on rat hippocampus and striatum extracellular lactate. *The American journal of physiology*. 1990;259(4 Pt 2):R773-9.

[93] Gómez-Pinilla, F., Dao, L., So, V. Physical exercise induces FGF-2 and its mRNA in the hippocampus. *Brain research*. 1997;764(1-2):1-8.

[94] Ickes, B. R., Pham, T. M., Sanders, L. A., Albeck, D. S., Mohammed, A. H., Granholm, A.-C. Long-Term Environmental Enrichment Leads to Regional Increases in Neurotrophin Levels in Rat Brain. *Experimental neurology*. 2000;164(1):45-52.

[95] Yoshida, Y., Goto, M., Tsutsui, J.-I., Ozawa, M., Sato, E., Osame, M., et al. Midkine is present in the early stage of cerebral infarct. *Developmental Brain Research*. 1995;85(1):25-30.

[96] Kermani, P., Hempstead, B. Brain-Derived Neurotrophic Factor: A Newly Described Mediator of Angiogenesis. *Trends Cardiovasc. Med.* 2007;17(4):140-3.

[97] Keiner, S., Witte, O. W., Redecker, C. Immunocytochemical detection of newly generated neurons in the perilesional area of cortical infarcts after intraventricular application of brain-derived neurotrophic factor. *J. Neuropathol. Exp. Neurol.* 2009;68(1):83-93.

[98] Schabitz, W. R., Steigleder, T., Cooper-Kuhn, C. M., Schwab, S., Sommer, C., Schneider, A., et al. Intravenous brain-derived neurotrophic factor enhances poststroke sensorimotor recovery and stimulates neurogenesis. *Stroke; a journal of cerebral circulation*. 2007;38(7): 2165-72.

[99] Waterhouse, E. G., Xu, B. New insights into the role of brain-derived neurotrophic factor in synaptic plasticity. *Molecular and Cellular Neuroscience*. 2009;42(2):81-9.

[100] Schäbitz, W. R., Schwab, S., Spranger, M., Hacke, W. Intraventricular brain-derived neurotrophic factor reduces infarct size after focal cerebral ischemia in rats. *J. Cereb. Blood Flow Metab.* 1997;17(5):500-6.

[101] Wu, D. Neuroprotection in experimental stroke with targeted neurotrophins. *NeuroRx: the journal of the American Society for Experimental NeuroTherapeutics*. 2005;2(1):120-8.

[102] Chen, A., Xiong, L. J., Tong, Y., Mao, M. The neuroprotective roles of BDNF in hypoxic ischemic brain injury. *Biomedical reports*. 2013;1 (2): 167-76.

[103] Madinier, A., Bertrand, N., Mossiat, C., Prigent-Tessier, A., Beley, A., Marie, C., et al. Microglial involvement in neuroplastic changes following focal brain ischemia in rats. *PloS one*. 2009;4(12):e8101.

[104] Kokaia, Z., Andsberg, G., Yan, Q., Lindvall, O. Rapid alterations of BDNF protein levels in the rat brain after focal ischemia: evidence for increased synthesis and anterograde axonal transport. *Experimental neurology*. 1998;154(2):289-301.

[105] Béjot, Y., Prigent-Tessier, A., Cachia, C., Giroud, M., Mossiat, C., Bertrand, N., et al. Time-dependent contribution of non neuronal cells to BDNF production after ischemic stroke in rats. *Neurochem. Int.* 2011; 58(1):102-11.

[106] Ding, Q., Ying, Z., Gomez-Pinilla, F. Exercise influences hippocampal plasticity by modulating brain-derived neurotrophic factor processing. *Neuroscience*. 2011;192:773-80.

[107] Vaynman, S., Ying, Z., Gomez-Pinilla, F. Hippocampal BDNF mediates the efficacy of exercise on synaptic plasticity and cognition. *The European journal of neuroscience*. 2004;20(10):2580-90.

[108] Brunet, A., Bonni, A., Zigmond, M. J., Lin, M. Z., Juo, P., Hu, L. S., et al. Akt promotes cell survival by phosphorylating and inhibiting a Forkhead transcription factor. *Cell*. 1999;96(6):857-68.

[109] Mitchell, A. C. Neuroprotection by physical activity. *Vanderbilt. Rev*. 2010;2:76-81.

[110] Wang, T., Xie, K., Lu, B. Neurotrophins promote maturation of developing neuromuscular synapses. *The Journal of neuroscience: the official journal of the Society for Neuroscience*. 1995;15(7 Pt 1):4796-805.

[111] Brock, T. O., O'Callaghan, J. P. Quantitative changes in the synaptic vesicle proteins synapsin I and p38 and the astrocyte-specific protein glial fibrillary acidic protein are associated with chemical-induced injury to the rat central nervous system. *The Journal of neuroscience: the official journal of the Society for Neuroscience*. 1987;7(4):931-42.

[112] Chen, J., Qin, J., Su, Q., Liu, Z., Yang, J. Treadmill rehabilitation treatment enhanced BDNF-TrkB but not NGF-TrkA signaling in a mouse intracerebral hemorrhage model. *Neurosci. Lett*. 2012;529(1):28-32.

[113] Hu, F. B., Stampfer, M. J., Colditz, G. A., Ascherio, A., Rexrode, K. M., Willett, W. C., et al. Physical activity and risk of stroke in women. *JAMA: the journal of the American Medical Association*. 2000;283 (22): 2961-7.

[114] Lee, I. M., Paffenbarger, R. S., Jr. Physical activity and stroke incidence: the Harvard Alumni Health Study. *Stroke; a journal of cerebral circulation*. 1998;29(10):2049-54.

[115] Laurin, D., Verreault, R., Lindsay, J., MacPherson, K., Rockwood, K. Physical activity and risk of cognitive impairment and dementia in elderly persons. *Archives of neurology*. 2001;58(3):498-504.

[116] van Praag, H., Christie, B. R., Sejnowski, T. J., Gage, F. H. Running enhances neurogenesis, learning, and long-term potentiation in mice. *Proceedings of the National Academy of Sciences of the United States of America*. 1999;96(23):13427-31.

[117] Fordyce, D. E., Wehner, J. M. Physical activity enhances spatial learning performance with an associated alteration in hippocampal protein kinase C activity in C57BL/6 and DBA/2 mice. *Brain research*. 1993;619(1-2): 111-9.

[118] Grealy, M. A., Johnson, D. A., Rushton, S. K. Improving cognitive function after brain injury: the use of exercise and virtual reality. *Archives of physical medicine and rehabilitation*. 1999;80(6):661-7.

[119] Neeper, S. A., Gomez-Pinilla, F., Choi, J., Cotman, C. W. Physical activity increases mRNA for brain-derived neurotrophic factor and nerve growth factor in rat brain. *Brain research*. 1996;726(1-2):49-56.

[120] Ploughman, M., Windle, V., MacLellan, C. L., White, N., Dore, J. J., Corbett, D. Brain-derived neurotrophic factor contributes to recovery of skilled reaching after focal ischemia in rats. *Stroke; a journal of cerebral circulation*. 2009;40(4):1490-5.

[121] Chen, M. J., Russo-Neustadt, A. A. Exercise activates the phosphatidylinositol 3-kinase pathway. *Brain research Molecular brain research*. 2005;135(1-2):181-93.

[122] Molteni, R., Ying, Z., Gomez-Pinilla, F. Differential effects of acute and chronic exercise on plasticity-related genes in the rat hippocampus revealed by microarray. *The European journal of neuroscience*. 2002; 16 (6):1107-16.

[123] Finkbeiner, S., Tavazoie, S. F., Maloratsky, A., Jacobs, K. M., Harris, K. M., Greenberg, M. E. CREB: A Major Mediator of Neuronal Neurotrophin Responses. *Neuron*. 1997;19(5):1031-47.

[124] Gottschalk, W. A., Jiang, H., Tartaglia, N., Feng, L., Figurov, A., Lu, B. Signaling mechanisms mediating BDNF modulation of synaptic plasticity in the hippocampus. *Learning and memory* (Cold Spring Harbor, NY). 1999;6(3):243-56.

[125] Hicks, A., Davis, S., Rodger, J., Helme-Guizon, A., Laroche, S., Mallet, J. Synapsin I and syntaxin 1B: key elements in the control of neurotransmitter release are regulated by neuronal activation and long-term potentiation in vivo. *Neuroscience*. 1997;79(2):329-40.

[126] Jovanovic, J. N., Czernik, A. J., Fienberg, A. A., Greengard, P., Sihra, T. S. Synapsins as mediators of BDNF-enhanced neurotransmitter release. *Nature neuroscience*. 2000;3(4):323-9.

[127] Abel, T., Kandel, E. Positive and negative regulatory mechanisms that mediate long-term memory storage. *Brain Research Reviews*. 1998;26 (2-3):360-78.

[128] Silva, A. J., Kogan, J. H., Frankland, P. W., Kida, S. CREB and memory. *Annual review of neuroscience* 1998. p. 127-48.
[129] Mårtensson, J., Eriksson, J., Bodammer, N. C., Lindgren, M., Johansson, M., Nyberg, L., et al. Growth of language-related brain areas after foreign language learning. *NeuroImage*. 2012;63(1):240-4.
[130] Warraich, Z., Kleim, J. A. Neural Plasticity: The Biological Substrate For Neurorehabilitation. *PM and R*. 2010;2(12, Supplement):S208-S19.
[131] Merzenich, M. M., Kaas, J. H., Wall, J., Nelson, R. J., Sur, M., Felleman, D. Topographic reorganization of somatosensory cortical areas 3b and 1 in adult monkeys following restricted deafferentation. *Neuroscience*. 1983;8(1):33-55.
[132] Brown, C. E., Aminoltejari, K., Erb, H., Winship, I. R., Murphy, T. H. In vivo voltage-sensitive dye imaging in adult mice reveals that somatosensory maps lost to stroke are replaced over weeks by new structural and functional circuits with prolonged modes of activation within both the peri-infarct zone and distant sites. *The Journal of neuroscience: the official journal of the Society for Neuroscience*. 2009; 29(6):1719-34.
[133] Lazarov, O., Robinson, J., Tang, Y. P., Hairston, I. S., Korade-Mirnics, Z., Lee, V. M., et al. Environmental enrichment reduces Abeta levels and amyloid deposition in transgenic mice. *Cell*. 2005;120(5):701-13.
[134] van Praag, H., Shubert, T., Zhao, C., Gage, F. H. Exercise enhances learning and hippocampal neurogenesis in aged mice. *The Journal of neuroscience: the official journal of the Society for Neuroscience*. 2005; 25(38):8680-5.
[135] Kuhn, H. G., Dickinson-Anson, H., Gage, F. H. Neurogenesis in the dentate gyrus of the adult rat: age-related decrease of neuronal progenitor proliferation. *The Journal of neuroscience: the official journal of the Society for Neuroscience*. 1996;16(6):2027-33.
[136] Heine, V. M., Maslam, S., Joels, M., Lucassen, P. J. Prominent decline of newborn cell proliferation, differentiation, and apoptosis in the aging dentate gyrus, in absence of an age-related hypothalamus-pituitary-adrenal axis activation. *Neurobiology of aging*. 2004;25(3):361-75.
[137] Altman, J., Das, G. D. Autoradiographic and histological evidence of postnatal hippocampal neurogenesis in rats. *The Journal of comparative neurology*. 1965;124(3):319-35.
[138] Eriksson, P. S., Perfilieva, E., Bjork-Eriksson, T., Alborn, A. M., Nordborg, C., Peterson, D. A., et al. Neurogenesis in the adult human hippocampus. *Nature medicine*. 1998;4(11):1313-7.

[139] Colcombe, S. J., Erickson, K. I., Raz, N., Webb, A. G., Cohen, N. J., McAuley, E., et al. Aerobic fitness reduces brain tissue loss in aging humans. *The journals of gerontology Series A, Biological sciences and medical sciences*. 2003;58(2):176-80.

[140] Jin, K., Wang, X., Xie, L., Mao, X. O., Zhu, W., Wang, Y., et al. Evidence for stroke-induced neurogenesis in the human brain. *Proceedings of the National Academy of Sciences of the United States of America*. 2006;103(35):13198-202.

[141] Zigova, T., Pencea, V., Wiegand, S. J., Luskin, M. B. Intraventricular administration of BDNF increases the number of newly generated neurons in the adult olfactory bulb. *Molecular and cellular neurosciences*. 1998;11(4):234-45.

[142] Pencea, V., Bingaman, K. D., Wiegand, S. J., Luskin, M. B. Infusion of brain-derived neurotrophic factor into the lateral ventricle of the adult rat leads to new neurons in the parenchyma of the striatum, septum, thalamus, and hypothalamus. *The Journal of neuroscience: the official journal of the Society for Neuroscience*. 2001;21(17):6706-17.

[143] Rossi, C., Angelucci, A., Costantin, L., Braschi, C., Mazzantini, M., Babbini, F., et al. Brain-derived neurotrophic factor (BDNF) is required for the enhancement of hippocampal neurogenesis following environmental enrichment. *The European journal of neuroscience*. 2006; 24(7):1850-6.

[144] Gomez-Pinilla, F., Dao, L., So, V. Physical exercise induces FGF-2 and its mRNA in the hippocampus. *Brain research*. 1997;764(1-2):1-8.

[145] van Praag, H. Neurogenesis and exercise: past and future directions. *Neuromolecular medicine*. 2008;10(2):128-40.

[146] Palmer, T. D., Willhoite, A. R., Gage, F. H. Vascular niche for adult hippocampal neurogenesis. *The Journal of comparative neurology*. 2000;425(4):479-94.

[147] Shen, Q., Goderie, S. K., Jin, L., Karanth, N., Sun, Y., Abramova, N., et al. Endothelial cells stimulate self-renewal and expand neurogenesis of neural stem cells. *Science* (New York, NY). 2004;304(5675):1338-40.

[148] Pereira, A. C., Huddleston, D. E., Brickman, A. M., Sosunov, A. A., Hen, R., McKhann, G. M., et al. An in vivo correlate of exercise-induced neurogenesis in the adult dentate gyrus. *Proceedings of the National Academy of Sciences of the United States of America*. 2007;104(13): 5638-43.

[149] Thored, P., Wood, J., Arvidsson, A., Cammenga, J., Kokaia, Z., Lindvall, O. Long-term neuroblast migration along blood vessels in an

area with transient angiogenesis and increased vascularization after stroke. *Stroke; a journal of cerebral circulation.* 2007;38(11):3032-9.

[150] Jin, K., Zhu, Y., Sun, Y., Mao, X. O., Xie, L., Greenberg, D. A. Vascular endothelial growth factor (VEGF) stimulates neurogenesis in vitro and in vivo. *Proceedings of the National Academy of Sciences of the United States of America.* 2002;99(18):11946-50.

[151] Cao, L., Jiao, X., Zuzga, D. S., Liu, Y., Fong, D. M., Young, D., et al. VEGF links hippocampal activity with neurogenesis, learning and memory. *Nature genetics.* 2004;36(8):827-35.

[152] Aberg, M. A., Aberg, N. D., Hedbacker, H., Oscarsson, J., Eriksson, P. S. Peripheral infusion of IGF-I selectively induces neurogenesis in the adult rat hippocampus. *The Journal of neuroscience: the official journal of the Society for Neuroscience.* 2000;20(8):2896-903.

[153] Lichtenwalner, R. J., Forbes, M. E., Bennett, S. A., Lynch, C. D., Sonntag, W. E., Riddle, D. R. Intracerebroventricular infusion of insulin-like growth factor-I ameliorates the age-related decline in hippocampal neurogenesis. *Neuroscience.* 2001;107(4):603-13.

[154] Greenberg, D. A. Angiogenesis and stroke. *Drug news and perspectives.* 1998;11(5):265-70.

[155] Black, J. E., Isaacs, K. R., Anderson, B. J., Alcantara, A. A., Greenough, W. T. Learning causes synaptogenesis, whereas motor activity causes angiogenesis, in cerebellar cortex of adult rats. *Proceedings of the National Academy of Sciences of the United States of America.* 1990; 87 (14):5568-72.

[156] Kleim, J. A., Cooper, N. R., VandenBerg, P. M. Exercise induces angiogenesis but does not alter movement representations within rat motor cortex. *Brain research.* 2002;934(1):1-6.

[157] Swain, R. A., Harris, A. B., Wiener, E. C., Dutka, M. V., Morris, H. D., Theien, B. E., et al. Prolonged exercise induces angiogenesis and increases cerebral blood volume in primary motor cortex of the rat. *Neuroscience.* 2003;117(4):1037-46.

[158] Anderson, B. J., Eckburg, P. B., Relucio, K. I. Alterations in the thickness of motor cortical subregions after motor-skill learning and exercise. *Learning and memory* (Cold Spring Harbor, NY). 2002;9(1):1-9.

[159] Ding, Q., Vaynman, S., Akhavan, M., Ying, Z., Gomez-Pinilla, F. Insulin-like growth factor I interfaces with brain-derived neurotrophic factor-mediated synaptic plasticity to modulate aspects of exercise-induced cognitive function. *Neuroscience.* 2006;140(3):823-33.

[160] Ding, Y. H., Li, J., Zhou, Y., Rafols, J. A., Clark, J. C., Ding, Y. Cerebral angiogenesis and expression of angiogenic factors in aging rats after exercise. *Current neurovascular research*. 2006;3(1):15-23.

[161] Carro, E., Nunez, A., Busiguina, S., Torres-Aleman, I. Circulating insulin-like growth factor I mediates effects of exercise on the brain. *The Journal of neuroscience: the official journal of the Society for Neuroscience*. 2000;20(8):2926-33.

[162] Fabel, K., Fabel, K., Tam, B., Kaufer, D., Baiker, A., Simmons, N., et al. VEGF is necessary for exercise-induced adult hippocampal neurogenesis. *The European journal of neuroscience*. 2003;18(10):2803-12.

[163] Trejo, J. L., Carro, E., Torres-Aleman, I. Circulating insulin-like growth factor I mediates exercise-induced increases in the number of new neurons in the adult hippocampus. *The Journal of neuroscience: the official journal of the Society for Neuroscience*. 2001;21(5):1628-34.

[164] Carmichael, S. T., Chesselet, M. F. Synchronous neuronal activity is a signal for axonal sprouting after cortical lesions in the adult. *The Journal of neuroscience: the official journal of the Society for Neuroscience*. 2002;22(14):6062-70.

[165] Dancause, N., Barbay, S., Frost, S. B., Plautz, E. J., Chen, D., Zoubina, E. V., et al. Extensive cortical rewiring after brain injury. *The Journal of neuroscience: the official journal of the Society for Neuroscience*. 2005; 25(44):10167-79.

[166] Brown, C. E., Li, P., Boyd, J. D., Delaney, K. R., Murphy, T. H. Extensive turnover of dendritic spines and vascular remodeling in cortical tissues recovering from stroke. *The Journal of neuroscience: the official journal of the Society for Neuroscience*. 2007;27(15):4101-9.

[167] Jones, T. A., Schallert, T. Use-dependent growth of pyramidal neurons after neocortical damage. *The Journal of neuroscience: the official journal of the Society for Neuroscience*. 1994;14(4):2140-52.

[168] Liauw, J., Hoang, S., Choi, M., Eroglu, C., Choi, M., Sun, G. H., et al. Thrombospondins 1 and 2 are necessary for synaptic plasticity and functional recovery after stroke. *Journal of cerebral blood flow and metabolism: official journal of the International Society of Cerebral Blood Flow and Metabolism*. 2008;28(10):1722-32.

[169] Carmichael, S. T., Archibeque, I., Luke, L., Nolan, T., Momiy, J., Li, S. Growth-associated gene expression after stroke: evidence for a growth-promoting region in peri-infarct cortex. *Experimental neurology*. 2005; 193(2):291-311.

[170] Stroemer, R. P., Kent, T. A., Hulsebosch, C. E. Neocortical neural sprouting, synaptogenesis, and behavioral recovery after neocortical infarction in rats. *Stroke; a journal of cerebral circulation*. 1995;26(11): 2135-44.

[171] Comelli, M. C., Guidolin, D., Seren, M. S., Zanoni, R., Canella, R., Rubini, R., et al. Time course, localization and pharmacological modulation of immediate early inducible genes, brain-derived neurotrophic factor and trkB messenger RNAs in the rat brain following photochemical stroke. *Neuroscience*. 1993;55(2):473-90.

[172] Cheatwood, J. L., Emerick, A. J., Schwab, M. E., Kartje, G. L. Nogo-A expression after focal ischemic stroke in the adult rat. *Stroke; a journal of cerebral circulation*. 2008;39(7):2091-8.

[173] Lee, J. K., Kim, J. E., Sivula, M., Strittmatter, S. M. Nogo receptor antagonism promotes stroke recovery by enhancing axonal plasticity. *The Journal of neuroscience: the official journal of the Society for Neuroscience*. 2004;24(27):6209-17.

[174] Papadopoulos, C. M., Tsai, S. Y., Cheatwood, J. L., Bollnow, M. R., Kolb, B. E., Schwab, M. E., et al. Dendritic plasticity in the adult rat following middle cerebral artery occlusion and Nogo-a neutralization. *Cerebral cortex* (New York, NY: 1991). 2006;16(4):529-36.

[175] Murphy, T. H., Corbett, D. Plasticity during stroke recovery: from synapse to behaviour. *Nat. Rev. Neurosci*. 2009;10(12):861-72.

[176] Hobohm, C., Gunther, A., Grosche, J., Rossner, S., Schneider, D., Bruckner, G. Decomposition and long-lasting downregulation of extracellular matrix in perineuronal nets induced by focal cerebral ischemia in rats. *Journal of neuroscience research*. 2005;80(4):539-48.

[177] Deguchi, K., Takaishi, M., Hayashi, T., Oohira, A., Nagotani, S., Li, F., et al. Expression of neurocan after transient middle cerebral artery occlusion in adult rat brain. *Brain research*. 2005;1037(1-2):194-9.

In: Exercise Training
Editor: Lucy Dukes

ISBN: 978-1-63463-501-1

Chapter 2

CONSUMER GOALS AND FOOD CONSUMPTION IN EXERCISE CONTEXTS

Joerg Koenigstorfer
Technische Universität München, Munich, Germany

ABSTRACT

The goal of this chapter is to review the importance of contextual exercise factors, such as a certain name of exercise bouts (e.g., "fat-burning") and a certain framing of exercise bouts (e.g., "enjoyable activity"), for food consumption depending on consumers' goal states. In an effort to follow a healthy lifestyle, individuals have various goals in mind. These goals are often incompatible to each other and therefore produce goal conflicts in individuals, such as the conflict between wanting to watch a movie with friends in the evening and wanting a fit body. Against the background of the increasing prevalence of overweight and obesity worldwide, this chapter specifically looks at goal conflicts of individuals that are at greatest risk of failing to achieve their long-term goals, such as self-imposed exercisers or dietary restrained eaters, and presents empirical evidence that contextual exercise references often rather harm (than help) vulnerable consumer groups attain desirable long-term health and fitness goals. The chapter discusses implications from the perspective of public health and product/service providers.

Introduction

Exercise is one component of daily energy expenditure in humans. It has become an important part of healthy lifestyles, because individuals are less active both at work and at home compared to earlier days and because today's environment makes it easy for individuals to be inactive, such as when people use elevators instead of stairs, cars instead of bicycles, and technology instead of activities with full body movement (e.g., online shopping versus shopping in stores; playing computer games versus playing ball games). Beside exercise, nutrition is another factor that is associated with healthy lifestyles. In industrialized countries, most individuals have complete control over both exercise and nutrition, that is, they can decide whether they exercise or not (and for how long they exercise and what the intensity is), and what (and how much) food they eat. During one typical week, individuals make thousands of these decisions, and the goals that individuals have in mind often guide them when making decisions, be them conscious or unconscious.

There is more and more evidence that the interactions between exercise and food consumption are not only driven by physiological factors, but that contextual factors that are present in the environment guide food consumption. The goal of this chapter is to review the importance of contextual exercise factors for (post-exercise) food consumption depending on consumers' goal states. In particular, the chapter looks at how much consumers eat after they have been exposed to contextual exercise factors (versus no exposure), such as a certain name and a certain framing of exercise bouts.

Interactions between Exercise and Food Consumption against the Background of Increasing Overweight and Obesity Rates

More and more individuals are interested in making food choices that are favorable for their personal health and well-being, as shown by a consumer survey of the IFIC Foundation (2010). At the same time, individuals are being offered food products that are considered or labeled as being "light" or "low-calorie" choices as well as "functional" options that generally claim to be beneficial to one's health and fitness. The consumer population has accepted these products (AC Nielsen, 2008) while, interestingly, average body weight and health problems have increased – not decreased (WHO, 2009). This can be partly explained by recent findings that contextual factors, such as labels, names, and claims related to health aspects, have the opposite of the intended effects and that they actually lead individuals to consume more in terms of calories – not less – on a single eating occasion (Wansink & Chandon, 2006). There is further evidence that overconsumption can also result from the presence of contextual exercise factors and that physiological factors (such as the need for energy) cannot explain these effects (Fenzl, Bartsch, & Koenigstorfer, 2014). Automatic associations that have been learned over time provide an explanation for this. In many cases, individuals are guided unconsciously by contextual references found in the environment without any volitional monitoring processes being involved (Laran & Janiszewski, 2009). The goals that individuals have in mind when they are exposed to contextual exercise factors influence how they respond to such stimuli. In what follows next, I will explain how goal conflicts provide explanations for exercise-nutrition interactions.

Consumer Goals and Conflicts

In an effort to follow a healthy lifestyle, individuals have various goals in mind. They thus make exercise and food decisions that are driven by multiple goals. These goals are often incompatible to each other and therefore produce goal conflicts in individuals, such as the conflict between wanting to watch a movie with friends in the evening and wanting a fit body as well as the conflict between wanting to eat tasty food when passing a bakery and wanting a slim body (Dhar & Simonson, 1999; Fishbach & Dhar, 2005; Stroebe, Mensink, Aarts, Schut, & Kruglanski, 2008). In order to solve such conflicts, individuals liberate themselves from attaining one goal versus another. Liberation describes the process when individuals free themselves from pursuing one goal over an incongruent goal; the progress that individuals make towards a focal goal (e.g., the health-related goal) then provides a justification to them for pursuing opposing goals, such as watching a movie with friends or eating tasty food (e.g., the enjoyment-related goals). However, not only actual, but even expected goal progresses can lead to moving away from an active health goal (Fishbach & Dhar, 2005; Fishbach, Friedman, & Kruglanski, 2003). Furthermore, the liberation mechanism can take place despite the fact that the focal health-related goal is actually not fulfilled (Wilcox, Vallen, Block, & Fitzsimons, 2009).

The concept of exercise (and related concepts, such as fitness, physical activity, and sports) is compatible with health-related goals, whereas it is (at least for most individuals) incompatible with enjoyment goals because it needs effort and time to become fit (Fishbach & Shah, 2006). The worldwide consensus regarding the benefits of physical activity for individuals' health is that people should be physically active on most, preferably all days of a week for at least 30 to 60 minutes at a moderate intensity (Haskell et al., 2007; USDA, 2005; WHO, 2003). Many individuals lack the time or the motivation to meet these guidelines. Nevertheless, being fit and active is a desirable goal for most individuals, and this is why contextual exercise factors interfere with the goals that individuals have in mind. For example, Crum and Langer (2007) found that room attendants in hotels who were informed that their work (cleaning hotel rooms) is good exercise and satisfies the Surgeon General's recommendations for an active lifestyle (versus control group) did not change their actual behavior, but, four weeks after the intervention, the participants of the informed group perceived themselves to be getting more exercise than before. In what follows next, I will briefly describe the results of the empirical studies that were conducted in the field of exercise-nutrition interactions (i.e., in connection with food consumption).

Goal Conflicts and Post-Exercise Food Consumption

Since this chapter looks at consumption in response to contextual exercise factors against the background of the increasing prevalence of overweight and obesity, this chapter specifically looks at goal conflicts of individuals who are at greatest risk of failing to achieve long-term goals. Those at greatest risk are consumers with low self-control, meaning that have a low ability to resist unhealthy foods that provide immediate rewards to them (Baumeister, 2002), and with high dietary restraint, meaning that individuals attempt to restrict their food intake. Low self-control consumers are more likely to be overweight or obese, and less likely to successfully lose weight (Crescioni et al., 2011). Restrained eaters are individuals who constantly worry about their weight and are chronically engaged in dieting efforts in order to achieve or maintain a desirable body weight (Herman & Mack, 1975). Also, those individuals are at greatest risk who self-impose physical activity – individuals with low behavioral regulation and high psychological distress, high fatigue levels, and low positive well-being when exercising – because they do not like to exercise and are prone to remain inactive throughout the day (Fenzl et al., 2014).

While there is only conceptual evidence for why low self-control and highly restrained eaters may be at risk of resolving goal conflicts in an unhealthful way (i.e., resulting in overconsumption), I will briefly present the results of one study that looked at the effects of contextual exercise factors on the tendency to overconsume in self-imposed exercisers. The study conducted by Fenzl et al. (2014) looked at the effects of the name of an exercise bout, in particular the name "fat-burning exercise" (as one specific contextual exercise reference), on post-exercise food consumption. The topic has high practical relevance, because many treadmills and bicycle ergometers offer fat-burning programs and because many health and fitness clubs offer fat-burning classes. These programs and classes are typically used to describe low-to-moderate intensity exercise bouts. There are reasons to believe that individuals perceive fat-burning exercise to be conducive to positive health and body appearance, including weight loss (Warburton, Nicol, & Bredin, 2006). First, individuals may believe that fat metabolism is stimulated, because the percentage of energy derived from burning fat (rather than carbohydrates or protein) is higher for less intense physical activity. An increase in fat metabolism is associated with several health benefits (Eriksson, Taimela, & Koivisto, 1997). Second, the concept of fat is closely linked to changes in energy balance (Wansink & Chandon, 2006). The fact that individuals burn off fat (and hence calories) may thus be more salient when they exercise using a fat-burning program than when the program is not explicitly labeled fat-burning.

Fenzl et al.'s (2014) study showed that self-imposed exercisers ate more food immediately after an exercise bout when the bout was labeled fat-burning exercise rather than endurance exercise. The fat-burning label acted as signal that fat metabolism has been activated, thus liberating individuals to consume more food after they have finished exercising. For these individuals exercising meant exerting self-control and resulted in the perception that a goal has been achieved, which made them more vulnerable to opposing goals, such as eating food after exercise (Fishbach & Dhar, 2005; Fishbach & Shah, 2006). In two laboratory studies, Werle, Wansink, and Payne (2014) showed that exercisers who perceived physical activity as fun (e.g., when it is labeled as a scenic walk rather than an exercise walk) consumed less dessert at mealtime and consumed fewer hedonic snacks on single eating occasions. They also present the results of a field study during a race that showed that the more fun athletes had during the race, the less likely they compensated with a hedonic snack afterwards.

The studies conducted by Fenzl et al. (2014) and Werle et al. (2014) provide evidence that contextual exercise factors, as part of actual exercise training, influence post-exercise food consumption. Today, many individuals are inactive. Yet, they are still exposed to exercise stimuli when making food decisions. In what follows next, I will briefly describe the results of empirical studies that looked at the effects of contextual exercise factors on food consumption, without any actual physical activity.

Is Actual Exercise Necessary to Influence Food Consumption?

Contextual reference to exercise (and related concepts, such as fitness, physical activity, and sports) exist in many forms, such as in the social environment (e.g., seeing a runner through the window while eating at McDonald's), in advertising (e.g., seeing an athlete as celebrity endorser [eventually for food] on television while sitting on the couch), and on the product packaging of the food (e.g., eating a cereal called "Fitness" for breakfast). In some cases, contextual exercise references may even indicate to individuals that eating the food will help them become fit (Koenigstorfer, Groeppel-Klein, Kettenbaum, & Klicker, 2013). Trail mix was used in the study conducted by Koenigstorfer et al. (2013) and the food was labeled either "Fitness" or "Trail Mix." The fitness food seemingly helped individuals achieve higher fitness levels and reduced the monitoring of food intake in these individuals. The contextual exercise references also made individuals feel less guilty after having consumed the food. Guilt is an "unpleasant emotional state associated with possible objections to [...] actions, inactions, circumstances, or intentions" (Baumeister, Stillwell, & Heatherton, 1994, p. 245). The presence of contextual exercise references on the food packaging reduced the tendency to feel guilty because the claim gave individuals a justification for consumption. Fitness cues on the food packaging also affected actual consumption volumes of foods (mediated by perceived serving size, that is, the intuitive belief how large a serving of the food is supposed to be) (Koenigstorfer et al., 2013).

There is further evidence that contextual exercise factors influence food consumption even though individuals are not physically active. In Fishbach and Dhar's (2005) study on liberating mechanisms, students expecting to work out stated higher intentions to have an indulging dinner compared with students who actually exercised. Werle, Wansink, and Payne (2011) showed that simply reading about physical activity can make consumers pour up to 59% more of snack foods into a bowl. In a laboratory setting, Albarracin, Wang, and Leeper (2009) observed a higher consumption volume of raisins after students had viewed exercise-related (vs. control) print advertisements.

Geyskens, Pandelaere, Dewitte, and Warlop (2007) showed that individuals who were primed supraliminally with health-related words (including fitness words) consumed more low-fat labeled food than consumers who were not primed with these words. They argued that individuals felt closer to the ideal weight in response to the priming. Applying these findings to food marketing practice, one can assume that contextual exercise factors increase consumption volumes (mostly independent of consumers' goal states). Exercise (and related concepts, such as fitness, physical activity, and sports) is associated with energy expenditure, and higher energy expenditure means that consumers can eat more to keep an isocaloric energy balance (or produce an energy deficit).

CONCLUSION

Political and consumer protection institutions aim to provide political and legal regulations that enable consumers to make reflected, well-informed and healthy food choices, thereby counteracting the increasing prevalence of overweight and obesity (e.g., BEUC, 2006; EC, 2005, 2009; USDA, 2005; WHO, 2004). High food consumption volumes during single eating occasions have been identified as one factor that drives the increasing prevalence of obesity. The author of this chapter has argued that food consumption volumes are not only influenced by physiological factors, but also by contextual factors. This is also true for post-exercise consumption volumes: There is both theoretical and empirical evidence that contextual exercise factors affect how much consumers eat during an eating occasion. The contextual factors do not only include one's own actual physical activity, but also physical activity names, labels, photos, and any other references to physical activity as part of the environment. In what follows next, I will briefly highlight some implications of the research findings, taking the perspective of both public health and product/service providers.

Post-Exercise Food Consumption

Self-imposing physical activity is a phenomenon that is often observed in individuals with body weight problems (Donovan & Penny, 2014). Based on the results of Fenzl et al.'s (2014) study, and from the public health perspective, it is recommended that exercise programs and classes are labeled in a way that consumers cannot form close connections with perceived goal fulfillment of fitness (in order to reduce liberation effects). Also, liberation-inducing labels (such as fat-burning names) may be made less salient during exercise in order to help reduce the overcompensation effect on immediate post-exercise food intake.

In addition to changing the labels given to exercise programs and classes and making them less salient, one might also recommend that health professionals in the field of exercise and nutrition attempt to strengthen the self-determination of individuals who are at greatest risk of being misled by contextual factors for certain exercise bouts. In the exercise domain, individuals are often told what is safe to do for them (and what is not safe), how hard and for how long they should work out; this is particularly true in exercise for weight management (Haskell et al., 2007). The results of Fenzl et al.'s (2014) and Werle et al.'s (2014) studies suggest that individuals should learn to consider physical activity as a rewarding and enjoyable activity and increase their ability to use internal factors to regulate behavior rather than relying on external, including social and societal motivating factors and pressures. Choosing a sport that matches the interest of the individual and which he or she will find enjoyable is one strategy that may help to achieve this goal. Manipulating how physical activity is framed can also increase self-determination. Werle et al. (2011 p. 335) stated that, "instead of describing [exercise] as a facilitation to weight loss, it can be presented as a critical way to tone one's self, strengthen bones, improve posture, and so forth." Use of such messages would emphasize that individuals make an active contribution to their health and well-being when they exercise, and that they determine their behavior and the resulting consequences by themselves. Van Kleef, Shimizu, and Wansink (2011) reported overcompensation and reduced motivation to exercise if individuals felt under pressure to do so or felt an obligation to exercise and to be fit and healthy. Product/service providers could improve the framing of physical activity – and perhaps avoid overconsumption effects – by including messages that increase self-determination and positive well-being and reduce stress and fatigue (Hills & Byrne, 2004).

Another recommendation is that individuals should learn to use physiological signals to infer the intensity of their exercise program rather than relying on contextual cues. Previous research has shown that promoting explicit knowledge is a difficult task in the exercise domain (Braham, Rosenberg, & Begley, 2012). This is particularly true when health practitioners prescribe physical activity (which is typically an indicator that an individual relies on external factors to carry out exercise); in these circumstances warning patients or clients about compensation is advisable, but may not be as effective as one might wish (King, 1999). Hills and Byrne (2004, p. 316) referred to previous research in their field (Hills & Byrne, 1998) when they wrote that "exercise prescription is both an art and a science." It can therefore be recommended that practitioners make physical activity prescriptions in such way that individuals are not tempted to feel – albeit implicitly – that they have attained desirable long-term goals such as attractive body appearance and low body weight because of the label attached to the form of exercise they have undertaken.

Fitness References on Food Packages

References to fitness are quite common in food products and are found in categories such as sweet and salty snacks (e.g., *Farmer*'s Fitness snack), drinks (e.g., *Powerade* Sports water), cereals (e.g., *Nestlé*'s Fitness cereal), packaged foods (e.g., *Knorr*'s Active soup), dairy products (e.g., *Müller*'s Fitness yogurt), breads (e.g., *Delba*'s Fitness bread), and spreads (e.g., *Fit & Aktiv* bread spread). These references can increase post-exercise food consumption. The product packaging makes individuals feel that they have become more fit despite the fact that they are not engaged in any actual physical activity while eating the food. One can argue that overconsumption is not in conflict with attaining health-related goals when the food product is considered to be healthful. However, maintaining or lowering one's body weight is an important goal to an estimated 72 percent of the U.S. population (Serdula et al., 1999). There is increasing evidence that individuals in developed countries struggle to maintain their energy balance, tending to consume more energy than they expend. In the long run, a positive energy balance causes weight gain, and weight gain is associated with several health risks (Pedersen, 2013).

From the public health perspective, agencies such as the Food and Drug Administration may educate consumers better about the interactions between physical activity cues and food intake, especially when consumers remain physically inactive. Also, agencies may evaluate the scientific evidence when food manufacturers make claims on the product packaging about fitness and food consumption. Cues that may be relevant for professional athletes may be irrelevant and misleading for persons that are mainly sedentary.

Concluding Remarks

I hope that this chapter inspires future research into the effects of contextual exercise factors on energy balance. While today's society has gathered good knowledge of what type of exercise (and how much) exercise produces positive health outcomes, we must gain a better understanding of when exercise references help (or harm) individuals achieve their long-term health goals (and when goal lapses occur).

References

AC Nielsen (2008). *Consumers and nutritional labeling – A global Nielsen report*, September. New York: AC Nielsen.

Albarracin, D., Wang, W., & Leeper J. (2009). Immediate increase in food intake following exercise messages. *Obesity*, *17*, 1451-1452.

Baumeister, R. F., Stillwell, A. M., & Heatherton, T. F. (1994). Guilt: An interpersonal approach. *Psychological Bulletin*, *115*, 243-267.

Baumeister, R. F. (2002). Yielding to temptation: Self-control failure, impulsive purchasing, and consumer behavior. *Journal of Consumer Research*, 28, 670-676.

BEUC (2006). *Discussion group on simplified labelling: Final report*. Brussels: Bureau Européen des Unions de Consommateurs.

Braham, R., Rosenberg, M., & Begley, B. (2012). Can we teach moderate intensity activity? Adult perception of moderate intensity walking. *Journal of Science and Medicine in Sport*, *15*, 322-326.

Crescioni, A. W., Ehrlinger, J., Alquist, J. L., Conlon, K. E., Baumeister, R. F., Schatschneider, C., & Dutton, G. R. (2011). High trait self-control predicts positive health behaviors and success in weight loss. *Journal of Health Psychology*, 16, 750-759.

Crum, A. J., & Langer, E. J. (2007). Mind-set matters: Exercise and the placebo effect. *Psychological Science*, 18, 165-171.

Dhar, R., & Simonson, I. (1999). Making complementary choices in consumption episodes: Highlighting versus balancing. *Journal of Marketing Research*, 36, 29-44.

Donovan, C. L., & Penny, R. (2014). In control of weight: The relationship between facets of control and weight restriction. *Eating Behaviors*, *15*, 144-150.

EC (2005). *Promoting healthy diets and physical activity: A European dimension for the prevention of overweight, obesity and chronic diseases*, Green Paper, COM(2005) 637 final. Brussels: Commission of the European Communities.

EC (2009). *EU platform on diet, physical activity and health*, Annual Report, May. Brussels: Commission of the European Communities.

Eriksson, J., Taimela, S., & Koivisto, V. A. (1997). Exercise and the metabolic syndrome. *Diabetologia*, *40*, 125-135.

Fenzl, N., Bartsch, K., & Koenigstorfer, J. (2014). Labeling exercise fat-burning increases post-exercise food consumption in self-imposed exercisers. *Appetite*, 81, 1-7.

Fishbach, A., & Dhar, R. (2005). Goals as excuses or guides: The liberating effect of perceived goal progress on choice. *Journal of Consumer Research*, *32*, 370-377.

Fishbach, A., & Shah, J. Y. (2006). Self-control in action: Implicit dispositions toward goals and away from temptations. *Journal of Personality and Social Psychology*, *90*, 820-832.

Fishbach, A., Friedman, R. S., & Kruglanski A. W. (2003). Leading us not into temptation: Momentary allurements elicit overriding goal activation. *Journal of Personality and Social Psychology*, *84*, 296-309.

Geyskens, K., Pandelaere, M., Dewitte, S., & Warlop, L. (2007). The backdoor to overconsumption: The effect of associating "low-fat" food with health references. *Journal of Public Policy and Marketing*, *26*, 118-125.

Haskell, W. L., Lee, I., Pate, R. R., Powell, K. E., Blair, S. N., Franklin, B. A., Macera, C. A., Heath, G. W., Thompson, P. D., & Bauman, A. (2007). Physical activity and public health: Updated recommendation for adults from the American College of Sports Medicine and the American Heart Association. *Medicine and Science in Sports and Exercise*, *39*, 1423-1434.

Herman, C. P., & Mack, D. (1975). Restrained and unrestrained eating. *Journal of Personality*, 43, 647-660.

Hills, A. P., & Byrne, N. M. (1998). Exercise prescription for weight management. *Proceedings of the Nutrition Society*, *57*, 93-103.

Hills, A. P., & Byrne, N. M. (2004). Physical activity in the management of obesity. *Clinics in Dermatology*, *22*, 315-318.

IFIC Foundation (2010). *2010 food & health survey: Consumer attitudes toward food safety, nutrition, & health*. Washington, DC: International Food Information Council Foundation.

King, N. A. (1999). What processes are involved in the appetite response to moderate increases in exercise-induced energy expenditure? *Proceedings of the Nutrition Society*, *58*, 107-113.

Koenigstorfer, J., Groeppel-Klein, A., Kettenbaum, M., & Klicker, K. (2013). Eat fit. Get big? How fitness cues influence food consumption volumes. *Appetite*, *65*, 165-169.

Laran, J., & Janiszewski, C. (2009). Behavioral consistency and inconsistency in the resolution of goal conflict. *Journal of Consumer Research*, *35*, 967-984.

Pedersen, S. D. (2013). Metabolic complications of obesity. *Clinical Endocrinology and Metabolism*, *27*, 179-193.

Serdula, M. K., Mokdad, A. H., Williamson, D. F., Galuska, D. A., Mendlein, J. M., & Heath, G. W. (1999). Prevalence of attempting weight loss and strategies for controlling weight. *Journal of the American Medical Association*, *282*, 1353-1358.

Stroebe, W., Mensink, W., Aarts, H., Schut, H., & Kruglanski, A. W. (2008). Why dieters fail: Testing the goal conflict model of cating. *Journal of Experimental Social Psychology*, *44*, 26-36.

USDA (2005). *Dietary guidelines for Americans* (6th ed.). Washington, DC: U.S. Department of Health and Human Services, U.S. Department of Agriculture.

Van Kleef, E., Shimizu, M., & Wansink, B. (2011). Food compensation: Do exercise ads change food intake? *International Journal of Behavioral Nutrition and Physical Acticity*, *8*, 661-664.

Wansink, B., & Chandon, P. (2006). Can "low-fat" nutrition labels lead to obesity? *Journal of Marketing Research*, *43*, 605-617.

Warburton, D. E., Nicol, C. W., & Bredin, S. S. (2006). Health benefits of physical activity: The evidence. *Canadian Medical Association Journal*, *174*, 801-809.

Werle, C. O., Wansink, B., & Payne, C. R. (2011). Just thinking about exercise makes me serve more food. Physical activity and calorie compensation. *Appetite*, *56*, 332-335.

Werle, C. O., Wansink, B., & Payne, C. R. (2014). Is it fun or exercise? The framing of physical activity biases subsequent snacking. *Marketing Letters*, doi: 10.1007/s11002-014-9301-6.

WHO (2003). *Diet, nutrition and the prevention of chronic diseases*, Technical Report Series 916. Geneva: World Health Organization.

WHO (2004). *Global strategy on diet, physical activity and health.* Geneva: World Health Organization.

WHO (2009). *Global database on Body Mass Index: An interactive surveillance tool for monitoring nutrition transition*. Geneva: World Health Organization.

Wilcox, K., Vallen, B., Block, L., & Fitzsimons, G. J. (2009). Vicarious goal fulfillment: When the mere presence of a healthy option leads to an ironically indulgent choice. *Journal of Consumer Research*, *36*, 380-393.

In: Exercise Training
Editor: Lucy Dukes
ISBN: 978-1-63463-501-1

Chapter 3

EXERCISE TRAINING IN CHRONIC NON-COMMUNICABLE DISEASES, PREVENTION AND HEALTH BENEFITS

Débora Tavares de Resende e Silva[1,*]***, Paola Ceratto***[2]***,***
Andréia Machado Cardoso[3]
and Margarete Dulce Bagatini[4]
Federal University Fronteira Sul, Brazil

ABSTRACT

The social and economic transformations which society has undergone since the last century have caused significant changes in morbidity and mortality in our population profile. Infectious and parasitic diseases, the leading causes of death in the beginning of last century, gave way to Chronic Non-Communicable Diseases (CNCDs). In 2008, the CNCDs were responsible for 63% of those occurring in the world and approximately 80% of these occur in low and middle income. The main causes of these diseases include modifiable risk factors such as smoking, harmful alcohol consumption, physical inactivity and unhealthy diet, and non-modifiable factors such as age, heredity, gender and race. Anti-inflammatory effects by reducing systemic levels of proinflammatory

* Corresponding author's email: Dra. Débora Tavares de Resende e Silva: deboratavares.silva@hotmail.com. Federal University Fronteira Sul, Rua General Osório, 413D. CEP: 89802-210. Caixa Postal 181. Bairro Jardim Itália, Chapecó, Santa Catarina, Brasil.

adipokines and changes in markers inflammation via the production of IL-6. Plasma levels of IL-6 increase exponentially during physical exercise and greater stimuli for its synthesis appears to be related to the decrease of glycogen content in muscle. Increased levels of intracellular calcium and increased formation of reactive oxygen species are also capable of activating the transcription factors that regulate the synthesis of IL-6. This increase in circulating IL-6 is responsible for a subsequent increase of circulating anti-inflammatory cytokines. Furthermore, most of these anti-inflammatory effects are secondary to decreased concentration of triglycerides in plasma and low density lipoprotein (LDL) and increasing the concentration of high density lipoprotein (HDL) generated by improved lipid profile induced by exercise, and another beneficial response to exercise is the syntax stimulation of endothelial nitric oxide. Research clearly demonstrate the effectiveness of exercise in preventing diseases, especially cardiovascular, thus increasing levels of physical activity has been shown to decrease mortality and all the different diseases worldwide causes. The guide recognizes the benefits of cardiovascular disease prevention, and encourages the promotion of health, wellness and fitness to the public in order to improve the overall quality of life of individuals. Research is need on the potential benefits of differential training as an approach to physical rehabilitation and exercise prescription could counteract the psychological effects of physical disease in different populations.

Chronic Non-communicable Diseases (CNCDs)

The social and economic transformations which society has undergone since the last century have caused significant changes in morbidity and mortality in our population profile. Infectious and parasitic diseases, the leading causes of death in the beginning of last century, gave way to Chronic Non-Communicable Diseases (CNCDs) (Brazil, 2008), characterized by not being transmitted by its long latency period, long-term evolution, irreversible damage and complications that cause varying degrees of disability or death (Married et al., 2009). Within this classification are cardiovascular diseases, their metabolic risk factors, certain types of cancers, lung disease and disability, currently the most important causes of morbidity and mortality (Terra et al., 2012; Rabbit et al., 2009; Brazil 2011).

In 2008, the CNCDs were responsible for 63% of those occurring in the world (Duncan et al., 2012) and approximately 80% of these occur in low and middle income. We have the example of Brazil, where CNCDs are the problem health of greater magnitude and correspond to 72% of the causes of deaths, strongly affecting the poor people and vulnerable groups (Brazil, 2011). The main causes of these diseases include modifiable risk factors such as smoking, harmful alcohol consumption, physical inactivity and unhealthy diet, and non-modifiable factors such as age, heredity, gender and race (Married et al., 2009). However, about 75% of them could be explained by two main factors, poor diet and physical inactivity (Coelho et al., 2009; Gleeson et al., 2011), which lead to the accumulation of visceral fat, accompanied by tissue infiltration Adipose by pro-inflammatory immune cells, developing a low-grade inflammatory state (Gleeson et al., 2011).

The CNCDs vary in severity: some are debilitating, disabling, and some other lethal. Affect many body systems and range from tooth decay, obesity, diabetes, hypertension, strokes, osteoporosis and cancer of many organs, as well as coronary heart disease. Recent research shows that it is possible, feasible and necessary a common dietary approach directed at prevention of common NCDs. The new epidemic of obesity, diabetes, osteoporosis, heart disease and lung, colon and rectum, breast, prostate and other cancers. This weight-multiplied disease is subject to become even worse as the Brazilian population increases and ages. Cannot be addressed only with medical and surgical treatments, although vitally important, but prevention treatments introduced in schools and community groups as nutritional education and change in life habits. Even in higher-income countries, the cost of treating NCDs constitute a huge social and economic burden. The models of care developed mainly by higher income countries refer almost exclusively to professionals in health interventions, such as mass screening, medical and surgical treatments available and palliative care, associated with the recommendation of behavioral changes and modes of life adopted by individuals (Brazil, 2012).

Anti-Inflammatory Effects of Exercise

Studies show that the responses promoted by non-strenuous exercise, especially continuously, prolonged (> 1.5 h) with intensity ranging from moderate to high (55 and 75% of O2 max), together with the reduction of overweight, exert several beneficial effects on several clinical and biochemical (Andrade et al., 2013; Terra et al., 2012; Henagan et al., 2012; Gleeson et al., 2011) parameters. The energy used by the body to perform the exercise is obtained by oxidation of muscle glycogen, blood glucose, and free fatty acids (FFA), triacylglycerol molecules stemmed (TG) of muscle tissue, adipose tissue, the plasma lipoproteins and a lower proportion of amino acids. One of the stages of energy production for the year is obtained by the hydrolysis (or lipolysis) that release of TG AG and glycerol. After hydrolysis the TG in the blood vessels, they are transported to the muscles, skeletal and cardiac, by albumin. FA in muscle cells are activated to acyl-CoA, and then transported by carnitine to the mitochondria where they are oxidized through the beta-oxidation process dependent on specific enzymes and transporter proteins that have increased their activity and with the passing of physical activity concentration providing more efficient use of lipids as an energy substrate (Bonifácio et al., 2005).

Physical training causes an increase in the rates of lipolysis and oxidation of TGM compared to TG stored in adipose tissue. One factor responsible for lipolysis is increased plasma concentrations of epinephrine, which activates beta-receptors of adipocytes. The molecules of FFA released during tissue lipolysis are not water-soluble and are transported in the blood by albumin (Bonifácio et al., 2005). The connection of the molecules of FFA to albumin causes there is a reduction of free albumin during exercise.

Recent studies have identified changes in the lipid profile and plasma lipoproteins in physically active individuals, observing lower concentration of total cholesterol, low density lipoprotein (LDL) and TG, increased high-density lipoprotein (HDL) as well as reduction subcutaneous adipose tissue (Bonifácio et al., 2005; Gleeson et al., 2011; Zelber-Sagi et al., 2014). It is also assumed that these beneficial changes in serum lipids decrease hepatic fat content, improving insulin sensitivity and glycemic control (Moningka et al., 2011), reducing the risk factors for the development of atherosclerosis and type II diabetes (Gleeson et al., 2011; Andrade et al., 2013; Ishikawa et al., 2012). Physiological changes produced by exercise promotes cardiovascular health, not only for the changes observed in the lipid profile, but also due to changes in the immune system, such as neuroendocrine mediators, release of steroids and the synthesis and production of proinflammatory cytokines such as the tumor necrosis factor alpha (TNF-α), IL-1β, which regulate the expression of selectins by endothelial cells, neutrophils attracted to the region, and IL-6 and IL-8 (Terra et al., 2012) cytokines.

IL-6 is a cytokine that participates in the inflammatory process and is considered a responsive interleukin inflammation. Acts as primary mediator of the acute phase response by stimulating the production of hepatic proteins, such as C-reactive protein (CRP) and protease inhibitors (e.g., protease inhibitor α-1), restricting the extent of inflammatory response by increasing synthesis of anti-inflammatory cytokines (Cruzat et al., 2007) such as IL-1ra and IL-10. This cytokine has been called miocina, since the contraction of skeletal muscles during prolonged exercise causes it to be released in high concentrations in the circulation (Terra et al., 2012). Increased synthesis and plasma levels of IL-6 during exercise is related to some factors such as the fall of the glycogen content in muscle, increased intracellular calcium levels and increased formation of reactive oxygen species, the which are able to activate the transcription factors that regulate the synthesis of IL-6. This increase in circulating IL-6 is responsible for a subsequent increase in circulating anti-inflammatory cytokines such as IL-10 and IL-1 receptor antagonist (IL-1ra), and including stimulating the release of cortisol from the adrenal glands and relative suppression of the expression of TNFa (Gleeson et al., 2011), PCR, and reduced expression of Toll like receptors (TLRs) on monocytes and macrophages (et al., 2010; Gleeson et al., 2011).

Decreased expression of Toll-like receptors (Toll-like receptor - TLRs) on macrophages and impaired antigen presentation to T cells, especially inflammatory prevents Th1, preventing tissue damage caused by inflammatory mediators and consequently reducing the risk of chronic inflammatory diseases. Besides its immunomodulatory effect, this miocina also has important metabolic effects, such as increased glucose uptake and fatty acid oxidation by skeletal muscle, increased hepatic gluconeogenesis and lipolysis in adipose tissue. In the same vein, the IL-8 miocina seems to exert angiogenic effects and IL-15, also produced by muscle contraction, seems to have anabolic effects and reduce adiposity (Terra et al., 2012).

The cytokines IL-6 and IL-8, secreted after tissue damage, stimulate the signaling pathway that activates the enzyme system nicotinamide adenine dinucleotide phosphate oxidase (NADPH) culminating with the release of reactive oxygen species (ROS) such as superoxide and hydroxyl radicals (Terra et al., 2012). Another also related to increased ROS during exercise factor is the high oxygen consumption by mitochondria during activity. The ROS molecules act as mitochondrial signaling to the cell, aiding in the adaptation to physical exercise, increasing the endogenous antioxidant capacity and insulin sensitivity through the expression of PGC reducing glucose metabolism, inducing mitochondrial metabolism and increases resistance to stress by induction of SOD (superoxide dismutase) 1, 2 and glutathione peroxidase, strategic defense enzymes EROS (Barbieri et al., 2013). Not limited to this, the EROS assist in acute regulation of cardiac contractility. It is known that excessive levels of ROS can modulate the activity of different proteins involved in coupling of excitation-contraction coupling, including the sarcoplasmic reticulum (SR) for releasing Ca2 +

channels, Ca2 + ATPase and the channel L-type Ca2 + (Noireaud, Andriantsitohaina, 2014).

Another exercise is beneficial response to blood pressure reduction, which involves physiological changes in various body systems. One of the mechanisms occurs through stimulation of endothelial nitric oxide synthase (eNOS or NOS III) (Moningka et al., 2011), found primarily in endothelial cell compartments called caveolae, which is responsible for the production of nitric oxide (NO), a vasoactive compound participating in the regulation of blood flow in different vascular beds including coronary blood flow, besides the essential importance for the maintenance of vascular tone (Dias et al., 2011). The production of nitric oxide is elevated during exercise due to increased blood flow, which results in prolongation of eNOS mRNA stability, increased eNOS protein and increased translation of NOS enzyme activity. Furthermore, the stress generated by cilhamento stimulates antioxidant extracellular superoxide mechanism. Because of stress-induced, cilhamento and up-regulation of eNOS and EC SOD have an improvement in endothelium-dependent vasodilation in parts of the circulation where blood flow is increased during exercise, such as skeletal muscle, pulmonary and coronary circulation, causing that the PA be at controlled levels (Moningka et al., 2011).

Another mechanism involved in the reduction of blood pressure during exercise is the activation of the sympathetic nervous system (SNS), which controls blood flow as detected physical effort. Occurs in two main ways, the first, the effort produced by exercise is constantly perceived by central command, however only elevates BP in detecting signs of maximum effort. Groups of sensory nerve fibers in skeletal muscle, which send afferent signals to the central nervous system to increase core flow when stimulated during exercise, mediate the second system. These sensory nerve endings include metaboreceptors, which are activated by ischemic metabolites generated during exercise, and mechanoreceptors, which are largely activated by mechanical stretch (Park et al., 2013) part.

However, the beneficial effects of physical activity are extremely large and some poorly understood. Recently has highlighted the improvement that exercise generates cognitive function, aiding in recovery from brain injury, reducing the risk of cognitive impairment associated with age and exerting antidepressant effects in depressed patients. Research has shown that exercise also increases the plasticity of the hippocampus, a key to cognitive and related to stress-related disorders, such as depression function structure. One aspect of the plasticity of the hippocampus that has received considerable attention is adult neurogenesis and the release of β-endorphin, which has been associated with cell proliferation and neuronal homeostatic balance, reflecting the cognitive and emotional conditions, and therefore a key factor for the beneficial effects of exercise (Koehl et al., 2008).

Although most biological mechanisms related to data generated by physical exercise are not yet fully understood, those already established become apparent association between physical activity and the promotion and restoration of health (Coelho et al., 2009; Cruzat et al., 2007, Smuder et al., 2011; Cassilhas et al., 2012; Barretti et al., 2012), improving the general health of people and delaying aging (Javadivala et al., 2013). In addition, there is a growing number of evidence showing an inverse association between physical activity and cardiovascular disease, including its metabolic risk factors (Rabbit et al., 2009; Moningka et al., 2011).

Indeed, exercise has been recognized as a non-pharmacological therapy of paramount importance in the prevention of several chronic diseases and their risk factors, including recommended as a first choice treatment for various health associations in the world (Zelber-Sagi et al., 2014; Gualano et al., 2011; Delbin et al., 2009; Silva et al., 2013; Cassilhas et al., 2012; Barretti et al., 2012; Ishikawa et al., 2012; Andrade et al., 2013), due to its ability to alleviate the symptoms of many of these conditions, making the exercise is increasingly cited and promoted as a therapeutic technique, hoping that the public be persuaded to participate in physical activities (Gleeson et al., 2011).

ROLE IN DISEASE PREVENTION AND HEALTH BENEFITS

Several biological mechanisms may be responsible for reducing the risk of chronic disease and premature death associated with routine physical activity. Since the routine physical activity appears to improve body composition (for example by the reduced abdominal obesity and improved weight control), improving lipoprotein lipid profile (for example, through triglycerides, increased reduction high density lipoprotein [HDL] cholesterol levels and decreased low-density lipoprotein [LDL] - to HDL ratios), improved glucose homeostasis and insulin sensitivity, reduce blood pressure, improve autonomic tone, reducing systemic inflammation; reducing blood clotting, improving coronary blood flow, improve cardiac function and improve endothelial function (Darren et al., 2009).

Since 1950s, physical inactivity is considered as a well-established risk factor for cardiovascular diseases (Morris & Crawford, 1958). A sedentary life style has a positive correlation with cardiovascular diseases development and increases more than two-fold the risk of chronic non-communicable diseases (CNCDs) (Boreaham & Riddoch, 2001; de Backer & de Backer, 2004; Prasad & Das, 2009). A vast body of evidence during the last few decades has shown the clear preventive role of physical activity in CNCDs (Prasad & Das, 2009).

Research clearly demonstrates the effectiveness of exercise in preventing diseases, especially cardiovascular, thus increasing levels of physical activity has been shown to decrease mortality and all the different diseases worldwide causes. Based on extensive evidence, recommendations for optimal levels of physical activity have been establish to promote and maintain health for everyone at different ages, so planned from childhood through adulthood and reaching seniors. Likewise, a strong research evidence established the efficacy and guidelines for physical activity to be perform and changes in behavior of the population was living was stimulated (Paffenbarger et al., 1986).

Primary prevention focuses on risk identification and modification of previous diseases in apparently healthy people, while secondary prevention aims to minimize and reverse the effects of established disease The American Physical Therapy Association (APTA) identified the value of disease prevention, with that The Guide to Physical Therapist Practice. The guide recognizes the benefits of cardiovascular disease prevention, and encourages the promotion of health, wellness and fitness to the public in order to improve the overall quality of life of individuals. Also, designate a preferred practice pattern "reduction/prevention primary risks for cardiovascular/pulmonary diseases", and indicates that, as part of the evaluation of any patient process, a physical therapist shall perform a review of the cardiopulmonary system that can include evaluation heart rate, blood pressure, respiratory rate, presence of edema (APTA, 2003).

Observational studies provide compelling evidence that regular physical activity and a high fitness level are associated with a reduced risk of premature death from any cause and from cardiovascular disease in particular among asymptomatic men and women. Furthermore, a dose-response relation appears to exist, such that people who have the highest levels of physical activity and fitness are at lowest risk of premature death.

Research is need on the potential benefits of differential training as an approach to physical rehabilitation and exercise prescription could counteract the psychological effects of physical disease in different populations. For example, increasing the complexity and variability of movement patterns in prescribing exercise programs can ease the effects of depression in populations not athletes and the physical effects of repetitive strain injuries experienced by athletes in elite sport programs and development. The range of benefits is because of different practices and aerobic or strengthening modalities that develop with each group or individual in particular (Schöllhorn et al., 2010).

Public Health organizations, such as American College of Sports Medicine (ACSM) and American Heart Association (AHA), have stated reports and recommendations for the promotion of physical activity to achieve health benefits and preventing diseases (Haskell et al., 2007). The mainly suggestion for adults is to exercise for 30 minutes at moderate-intensity levels on most, if not all, days of the week to achieve a weekly energy expenditure of at least 1,000 kcal. Low-intensity exercise should be performed more frequently and for longer duration (Haskell et al., 2007). However, increasing evidences about the different exercise protocols have emerging and suggesting an important role of interval training as well as straight training in improving cardiovascular health (Fagard, 2006; Collier et al., 2008; Grant et al., 2004; Fagard & Cornelissen, 2007; Banz et al., 2003; Ho et al., 2011; Figueroa et al., 2011).

Hypertension is linked to diabetes and metabolic diseases. Moreover is the pathology considered as the main cause of fatal cardiovascular diseases and exercise has been prescribed as the most important non-medical coadjutant in hypertension treatment (Pedersen, 2006; Hansen et al., 2010; Pal et al., 2013). It has become increasingly clear that independently of the exercise type, it will be able to trigger cardiovascular benefits. However, the performance improvement triggered by exercise practice rapidly decreases after a small resting period (about one month), thus, it should be practiced regularly to maintain the cardioprotector effects.

The considerations raised in the last researches about the exercises protocols suggest just little differences. Regarding to blood pressure improvement, aerobic exercise (30-40 minutes of training at 60%-85% of predicted maximal heart rate) most days of the week as well as resistance training (three sets of 10 repetitions at 10RM, three days a week) showed similar benefits, with most studies finding aerobic exercise to have more consistent effects (Fagard, 2006; Collier et al., 2008; Grant et al., 2004; Fagard & Cornelissen, 2007; Banz et al., 2003; Ho et al., 2011; Figueroa et al., 2011).

The information available about the impact of physical training in vascular function indicates that aerobic exercise (30-40 minutes at 65% of VO2 max) three times a week significantly reduce arterial stiffness, improve carotid artery compliance, and can restore vascular endothelial function in adults. Resistance exercise (four sets of 8–12 repetitions at 10 RM) and combination exercise training (15 minutes of aerobic and 15 minutes of resistance) 5 days a week also displayed improvement in vascular function (Goldberg et al., 2012;

Ferrier et al., 2001; Umpierre & Stein, 2007; Cook et al., 2006; Casey et al., 2007). Despite of the very well characterized benefits of continuous moderate exercise, the high-intensity interval training (HIT) has emerging as a novel proposal to prevent diseases and promotes health. Recently, Kessler et al. (2014) compared several studies using HIT and showed that this new exercise approach may result in a superior or equal improvement in fitness and cardiovascular health when compared to continuous exercise. The premise of using HIT in both healthy and clinical populations is that the vigorous activity segments promote greater adaptations via increased cellular stress, yet their short length, and the ensuing recovery intervals, allow even untrained individuals to work harder than would otherwise be possible at steady-state intensity (Roxburg et al., 2014; Kuehnbaum et al., 2014; Falcone et al., 2014). Additionally, HIT has been shown to be safe and effective in patients with a range of cardiac and metabolic dysfunction (Kessler et al., 2014).

It has been extensively proven that exercise reduces cardiovascular risk in subjects with diabetes, metabolic syndrome, coronary heart disease and hypertension, as well as in healthy people. Regular exercise training prevents disease and improves health through its beneficial effects to the cardiac and metabolic functions (Hansen et al., 2010; Pal et al., 2013). This occurs due to several mechanisms, including the improvement in skeletal muscle work capacity and antioxidant defenses, anti-inflammatory proprieties, reduction in resistance (thus, increasing conductance in the peripheral circulation), modulation of endothelial functions, among others (Gleeson et al., 2011; Pinto et al., 2012; Huang et al., 2013). CNCDs have a strong association to a pro-oxidant and pro-inflammatory status, which can be both causes and/or consequences of these pathologies. In these two points, a wide range of studies in both humans and animal models, have highlighted the beneficial effects of exercise (White et al., 2010; Pedersen, 2006; Pedersen, 2011; Gleeson et al., 2011; Cooper et al., 2002; Bloomer et al., 2004; Teixeira-Lemos et al., 2011; Cardoso et al., 2012).

Currently, it is well known that regular practice of exercises ameliorates the oxidative homeostasis of cells and tissues, by decreasing the basal levels of oxidative damage and increasing resistance to oxidative stress (Cooper et al., 2002; Bloomer et al.). Oxidative stress is one of the main consequences of exercise that prevents cell damage. This improvement in the oxidative status is related to prevention and treatment of CNCDs, such as hypertension and diabetes (Pedersen, 2006; Hansen et al., 2010; Teixeira-Lemos et al., 2011; Cardoso et al., 2012). Moreover, recent data regarding to the effects of exercise in the endothelial functions showed that physical active life style might reduce the inflammation in 70%. Additionally, there is a negative correlation between blood pressure and classic inflammatory markers (Skrypnik et al., 2014; Ryan et al., 2014). It is interesting to address that the beneficial effects from exercise will be achieved chronically, due to body metabolic adaptations related to each acute bout of exercise. However, during the acute exercise practice, that is, during a single bout of exercise, the organism is submitted to a stressful state (Di Meo et al., 2001; Huang et al., 2013). This state is linked to a harmful environment, triggered by a pro-inflammatory and pro-oxidant status (Gomes et al., 2012; Pedersen, 2011; Gleeson et al., 2011; Cardoso et al., 2012b; Cardoso et al., 2014). In the moment of the exercise, metabolic alterations due to increased body-working demand and oxygen consumption occurs, which will be intensity-dependents. These alterations will result in a high production of reactive oxygen species, culminating in oxidative stress and cell damage (Jackson et al., 2000). The oxidative stress related to acute exercise is also linked to the high production of pro-inflammatory cytokines, especially IL-6 (Daly et al., 2014; Skrypnik et al., 2014; Gleeson et al., 2011; Slattery et al., 2014). These apparently harmful effects of the acute exercise are necessary to the adaptations which will results an enhancement in oxidative and anti-inflamatory responses. Such responses will triggered improvement in cardiovascular and metabolic functions of the organism in both healthy and CNCDs patients (White et al., 2010; Pedersen, 2006; Pedersen, 2011; Gleeson et al., 2011).

Physical Fitness

Physical fitness is related to a physiological state of well-being, and is related to health and involves the components of physical fitness related to health, including cardiovascular fitness, musculoskeletal fitness, body composition and metabolism. In large epidemiological investigations, physical activity and physical fitness are often used interchangeably, with fitness commonly being treated as a measure of physical activity most accurate (albeit indirect). Physical fitness seems to be similar to physical activity in their relation to morbidity and mortality, but is more strongly predictive of health outcomes than physical activity (Erikssen, 2001; Myers et al., 2004). However, physical activity and fitness are strong predictors of risk of death to obtain accurate estimates of physical activity, many fitness consultants have primary (criterion and "gold") standards for measuring energy expenditure, such as direct observation motion or, in the laboratory, the technique of doubly labeled water or indirect in practical terms, however, the measures of physical activity and energy expenditure are obtained using heart rate monitors and motion sensors (pedometers and accelerometers). The assessment of physical fitness is often not feasible or practical in large population-based investigations. Fortunately, these studies have consistently shown an inverse gradient of health risk among groups of self-reported physical activity. From a public health perspective, Blair and colleagues have argued that it is preferable to encourage people to become more physically active instead of becoming physically fit, since, as they said, sedentary people probably achieve the latter if they do the first (Williams, 2001).

Musculoskeletal Fitness

Improvements in health status can occur as a result of a possible increase levels of physical activity, or in the absence of changes in aerobic fitness. This is evidenced in elderly populations where regular physical activity can lead to reductions in risk factors for chronic diseases and conditions of movement, beyond the disability without significantly changing the traditional markers of physiological performance (e.g., cardiac output and potential oxidative) and there are reports that physical activity routine can improve musculoskeletal fitness. There are studies showing that increased skeletal muscle fitness is associated with an improvement in the general health and reduction of disease risk. Some research found that the change of focus in research related to the health benefits of activities that overload the musculoskeletal system, and has been found that for older people, the ability to maintain functional independence is maintained in those who practice some activity physics. In fact, many activities of daily life do not require a great aerobic production, but rely on one or more of the components of musculoskeletal fitness (Warburton et al., 2001).

Definition of Terms

Physical Activity

Physical activity is defined as any bodily movement produced by skeletal muscles that require energy expenditure. Regular moderate intensity physical activity, such as walking, cycling, or participating in sports has significant benefits for health. For instance, it can reduce the risk of cardiovascular diseases, diabetes, colon and breast cancer, and depression. Moreover, adequate levels of physical activity will decrease the risk of a hip or vertebral fracture and help control weight.

Physical Fitness

Physical fitness is a general state of health and well-being or specifically the ability to perform aspects of sports or occupations. Physical fitness is generally achieved through correct nutrition, exercise, hygiene and rest. It is a set of attributes or characteristics that people have or achieve that relates to the ability to perform physical activity.

Physical Exercise

Physical exercise is any bodily activity that enhances or maintains physical fitness and overall health and wellness. It is performed for various reasons including strengthening muscles and the cardiovascular system, honing athletic skills, weight loss or maintenance, as well as for the purpose of enjoyment. Frequent and regular physical exercise boosts the immune system, and helps prevent the "diseases of affluence" such as heart disease, cardiovascular disease, Type 2 diabetes and obesity.

Conclusion

There appears to be a linear relation between physical activity and health status, such that a further increase in physical activity and fitness will lead to additional improvements in health status. There are enough reports to support the results that physical activity when practiced regularly contributes to primary and secondary prevention of several chronic diseases and is associated with a reduced risk of premature death. Studies show that there seems to be a relationship between quantity and regularity in physical activity with health status, such that the most physically active people are at lower risk. People who engage in exercise in excess of the levels recommended in the guidelines tend to gain more health benefits. Health promotion programs should guide people of all ages, since the risk of chronic disease begins in childhood and increases with age.

Taking this into account, to reach the desirable benefits from training, intensity, volume, and frequency of exercise should be careful programmed and the resting periods should receive special attention. If after some periods of intense activity the body does not recovery and restore the redox balance, it will undergoing to an undesirable state called overtraining, which, in addition to specific signs of metabolic fatigue, induces severe neuroendocrine disorders (Angeli et al., 2004). Thus, despite of the widely recognized benefits arising from regular practice of exercise, more research is need to define specific training programs related to each CNCDs.

References

Angeli A., Minetto M., Dovio A., Paccotti P. The overtraining syndrome in athletes: a stress-related disorder. *J Endocrinol Invest* 2004; 27: 603-612.

American Physical Therapy Association (APTA). *Guide to Physical Therapist Practice.* 2nd. Alexandria, VA: APTA; 2003.

Andrade, Geisielle Pereira; Cintra, Mariana MolinarMauad; Alves, Polyanna Miranda; Neto, Octavio Barbosa; Silva, Renata Calciolari Rossi e; SILVA, Valdo Jose Dias da; REIS, Marlene Antonia dos; ABATE, Débora Tavares de Resende e Silva; Remodeling of elastic layer of aorticartery after training by swimming in spontaneously hypertensive rats. *Experimental Biology and Medicine,* 2013.

Banz W. J., Maher M. A., Thompson W. G., Bassett D. R., Moore W., Ashraf M., et al. Effects of resistance versus aerobic training on coronary artery disease risk factors. *Exp Biol Med* (Maywood) 2003; 228: 434-40.

Barbieri, Elena; Sestili, Piero; Vallorani, Luciana et al. Mitohormesis in muscle cells: A morphological, molecular, and proteomic approach. *Muscles, Ligaments and Tendons Journal* 2013; 3 (4): 254-266.

Barretti, Diego Lopes Mendes; Magalhaes, Flavio de Castro; Fernandes, Tiago; Carmo, Everton Crivoi do; Rosa, Kaleizu Teodoro; Irigoyen, Maria Claudia; Negrao, Carlos Eduardo; Oliveira, Edilamar Menezes; Effects of Aerobic Exercise Training on Cardiac Renin Angiotens in System in an Obese Zucker Rat Strain. *PLoS ONE* 7(10), 2012.

Bloomer R. J., Goldfarb A. H.: Anaerobic exercise and oxidative stress: a review. *Can J Appl Physiol* 2004, 29(3):245-263.

Boreham C., Riddoch C. The physical activity, fitness and health of children. *J Sports Sci* 2001; 19:915-29.

Böhm, Joseane; Monteiro, Mariane Borba; Thomé, Fernando Saldanha; Efeitos do exercício aeróbio durante a hemodiálise em pacientes com doença renal crônica: uma revisão da literatura. *J Bras Nefrol* 2012; 34(2):189-194.

Bonifácio, N. P.; César, T. B. Metabolismo dos lípides durante o exercicio físico. *R. bras. Ci e Mov.* 2005; 13(4): 101-106.

Brasil. Ministério da Saúde. Secretaria de Vigilância em Saúde. Departamento de Análise de Situação de Saúde. *Plano de ações estratégicas para o enfrentamento das doenças crônicas não transmissíveis (DCNT) no Brasil 2011-2022*/Ministério da Saúde. Secretaria de Vigilância em Saúde. Departamento de Análise de Situação de Saúde. - Brasília: Ministério da Saúde, 2011.

Cardoso A. M., Abdalla F. H., Bagatini M. D., Martins C. C., Fiorin Fda S., Baldissarelli J., Costa P., Mello F. F., Fiorenza A. M., Serres J. D., Gonçalves J. F., Chaves H., Royes L. F., Belló-Klein A., Morsch V. M., Schetinger M. R. Swimming training prevents alterations in acetylcholinesterase and butyrylcholinesterase activities in hypertensive rats. *Am J Hypertens.* 2014 Apr; 27(4):522-9.

Cardoso A. M., Martins C. C., Fiorin Fda S., Schmatz R., Abdalla F. H., Gutierres J., Zanini D., Fiorenza A. M., Stefanello N., Serres J. D., Carvalho F., Castro V. P., Mazzanti C. M., Royes L. F., Belló-Klein A., Goularte J. F., Morsch V. M., Bagatini M. D., Schetinger M. R. Physical training prevents oxidative stress in L-NAME-induced hypertension rats. *Cell Biochem Funct.* 2013 Mar; 31(2):136-51.

Cardoso, A. M.; Bagatini M. D., Roth M. A., Martins C. C., Rezer J. F. P., Mello F. F., Lopes L. F. D., Morsch V. M. and Schetinger M. R. C. Acute effects of resistance exercise and intermittent intense aerobic exercise on blood cell count and oxidative stress in trained middle-aged women. *Braz J Med Biol Res,* December 2012, Volume 45(12) 1172-1182.

Casado, Letícia; Vianna, Lucia Marques; Thuler, Luiz Claudio Santos. Fatores de risco para Doenças Crônicas não Transmissíveis no Brasil: Uma revisão sistemática. *Revista Brasileira de Cancerologia,* 2009.

Casey D. P., Pierce G. L., Howe K. S., Mering M. C., Braith R. W. Effect of resistance training on arterial wave reflection and brachial artery reactivity in normotensive postmenopausal women. *Eur J Appl Physiol* 2007; 100: 403-8.

Cassilhas, R. C.; Lee, K. S.; Venâncio, D. P.; Oliveira, M. G. M.; Tufik, S.; Mello, M. T. de.; Resistanceexercise improves hippocampus-dependent memory. *Brazilian Journal of Medical and Biological Research*, Volume 45(12), 2012.

Coelho, Christianne de Faria; Burini, Roberto Carlos; Atividade física para prevenção e tratamento das doenças crônicas não transmissíveis e da incapacidade funcional. *Rev. Nutr.*, 2009.

Collier S. R., Kanaley J. A., Carhart R. Jr., Frechette V., Tobin M. M., Hall A. K., et al. Effect of 4 weeks of aerobic or resistance exercise training on arterial stiffness, blood flow and blood pressure in pre- and stage-1 hypertensives. *J Hum Hypertens* 2008; 22:678-86.

Cook J. N., Devan A. E., Schleifer J. L., Anton M. M., Cortez-Cooper M., Tanaka H. Arterial compliance of rowers: implications for combined aerobic and strength training on arterial elasticity. *Am J Physiol Heart Circ Physiol* 2006; 209: H1596-600.

Cooper C. E., Vollaard N. B., Choueiri T., Wilson M. T: Exercise, free radicals and oxidative stress. *Biochem Soc Trans* 2002, 30(2):280-285.

Cruzat, Vinicius Fernandes; Rogero, Marcelo Macedo; Borges, Maria Carolina; Tirapegui Julio; Aspectos atuais sobre estresse oxidativo, exercícios físicos e suplementação. *Rev Bras Med Esporte.* Vol. 13, N° 5 - Set/Out, 2007.

Daly, R. M.; O'Connell, S. L.; Mundell, N. L.; Grimes, C. A.; Dunstan, D. W.; Nowson, C. A. Protein-enriched diet, with the use of lean red meat, combined with progressive resistance training enhances lean tissue mass and muscle strength and reduces circulating IL-6 concentrations in elderly women: a cluster randomized controlled trial. *American Journal of Clinical Nutrition*, v. 99(4), p. 899-910, 2014.

Darren E. R. W., Crystal W. N.; Shannon S. D. B. Health benefits of physical activity: The evidence. *BMJ* 2009; 338: b688.

Delbin, Maria Andréia; Antunes, Edson; Zanesco, Angelina. Papel do exercício físico na isquemia/reperfusão pulmonar e resposta inflamatória. *Rev Bras Cir Cardiovasc.*, 2009.

De Backer G. G., De Bacquer D. Be physically active: The best buy in promoting heart health. *Eur Heart J* 2004; 25:2183-4.

Di Meo S., Venditti P: Mitochondria in exercise-induced oxidative stress. *Biol Signals Recept* 2001, 10(1-2):125-140.

Dias, Rodrigo Gonçalves; NEGRÃO, Carlos Eduardo; KRIEGER, Marta Helena; Óxido Nítrico e Sistema Cardiovascular: Ativação Celular,

Reatividade Vascular e Variante Genética. *Arq Bras Cardiol* 2011; 96(1): 68-75.

Duncan, B. B.; Chor, D.; Aquino, E. M. L. Doenças Crônicas Não Transmissíveis no Brasil: prioridade para enfrentamento e investigação. *Rev Saúde Pública*, 2012.

Erikssen G. Physical fitness and changes in mortality: The survival of the fittest. *Sports Med* 2001; 31:571-6.

Fagard R. H., Cornelissen V. A. Effect of exercise on blood pressure control in hypertensive patients. *Eur J Cardiovasc Prev Rehabil* 2007; 14:12-7.

Fagard R. H. Exercise is good for your blood pressure: effects of endurance training and resistance training. *Clin Exp Pharmacol Physiol* 2006; 33: 853-6.

Falcone P. H., Tai C. Y., Carson L. R., Joy J. M., Mosman M. M., McCann T. R., Crona K. P., Kim M. P., Moon J. R. Caloric expenditure of aerobic, resistance or combined high-intensity interval training using a hydraulic resistance system in healthy men. *J Strength Cond Res.* 2014 Aug 26. [Epub ahead of print].

Ferrier K. E., Waddell T. K., Gatzka C. D., Cameron J. D., Dart A. M., Kingwell B. A. Aerobic exercise training does not modify large-artery compliance in isolated systolic hypertension. *Hypertension* 2001; 38: 222-6.

Figueroa A., Park S. Y., Seo D. Y., Sanchez-Gonzalez M. A., Baek Y. H. Combined resistance and endurance exercise training improves arterial stiffness, blood pressure, and muscle strength in postmenopausal women. *Menopause* 2011; 18:980-4.

Gleeson, Michael; Bishop, Nicolette C.; Stensel, David J.; Lindley, Martin R.; Mastana, Sarabjit S.; NIMMO Myra A.; The anti-inflammatory effects of exercise: mechanisms and implications for the prevention and treatment of disease. *Nature Reviews/Immunology,* Vol. 11, 2011.

Gligoroska, Jasmina Pluncevic; Manchevska, Sanja; The Effect of Physical Activity on Cognition - Physiological Mechanisms. *Mat Soc Med.,* 24(3): 198-202, 2012.

Goldberg M. J., Boutcher S. H., Boutcher Y. N. The effect of 4 weeks of aerobic exercise on vascular and baroreflex function of young men with a family history of hypertension. *J Hum Hypertens* 2012; 26:644-9.

Gomes E. C., Silva A. N., De Oliveira M. R. Oxidants, antioxidants, and the beneficial roles of exercise-induced production of reactive species. *Oxid Med Cell Longev.* 2012; 2012:756132. doi: 10.1155/2012/756132. Epub 2012 Jun 3.

Grant S., Todd K., Aitchison T. C., Kelly P., Stoddart D. The effects of a 12-week group exercise programme on physiological and psychological variables and function in overweight women. *Public Health* 2004; 118: 31-42.

Gualano, Bruno; Pinto, Ana Lúcia de Sá; Perondi, Maria Beatriz; Roschel, Hamilton; Sallum, Adriana Maluf Elias; Hayashi, Ana Paula Tanaka; Solis, Marina Yazigi; Silva, Clóvis Artur. Efeitos terapêuticos do treinamento físico em pacientes com doenças reumatológicas pediátricas. *Rev Bras Reumatol.*, 2011.

Hansen D., Dendale P., van Loon L. J., Meeusen R. The impact of training modalities on the clinical benefits of exercise intervention in patients with cardiovascular disease risk or type 2 diabetes mellitus. *Sports Med.* 2010 Nov 1; 40(11):921-40. doi: 10.2165/11535930-000000000-00000.

Haskell W. L., Lee I. M., Pate R. R., Powell K. E., Blair S. N., Franklin B. A., Macera C. A., Heath G. W., Thompson P. D., Bauman A; American College of Sports Medicine; American Heart Association. Physical activity and public health: updated recommendation for adults from the American College of Sports Medicine and the American Heart Association. *Circulation.* 2007 Aug 28; 116(9):1081-93. Epub 2007.

Henagan, Tara M.; Forney, Laura; Dietrich, Marilyn A.; Harrell, Brian R.; Stewart, Laura K.; Melanocortin receptor expression is associated with reduced CRP in responde to resistance training. *J Appl Physiol*, 2012.

Ho S. S., Dhaliwal S. S., Hills A., Pal S. Acute exercise improves postprandial cardiovascular risk factors in overweight and obese individuals. *Atherosclerosis* 2011; 214:178-84.

Huang C. J., Webb H. E., Zourdos M. C., Acevedo E. O. Cardiovascular reactivity, stress, and physical activity. *Front Physiol.* 2013 Nov7; 4:314. doi: 10.3389/fphys.2013.00314.

Kessler H. S., Sisson S. B., Short K. R. The potential for high-intensity interval training to reduce cardiometabolic disease risk. *Sports Med.* 2014 Jun 1; 42(6):489-509. doi: 10.2165/11630910-000000000-00000.

Kuehnbaum N. L., Gillen J. B., Gibala M. J., Britz-Mckibbin P. Personalized metabolomics for predicting glucose tolerance changes in sedentary women after high-intensity interval training. *Sci Rep.* 2014 Aug 28; 4: 6166. doi: 10.1038/srep06166.

Ishikawa, Yuji; Gohda, Tomohito; Tanimoto, Mitsuo; Omote, Keisuke; Furukawa, Masako; Yamaguchi, Saori; Murakoshi, Maki; Hagiwara, Shinji; Horikoshi, Satoshi; Funabiki, Kazuhiko; Tomino, Yasuhiko; Effect of Exercise on Kidney Function, Oxidative Stress, and Inflammation in Type 2 Diabetic KK-AyMice. *Experimental Diabetes Research,* 2012.

Javadivala, Zeinab; Kousha, Ahmad; Allahverdipour, Hamid; Jafarabadi, Mohammad Asghari; Tallebian, Hossein; Modeling the Relationship between Physical Activity and Quality of Life in Menopausal-aged Women: A Cross-sectional Study. *Journal of Research in Health Sciences,* 2013.

Koehl, M.; Meerlo, P.; Gonzales, D.; Rontal, A.; Turek, F. W.; Abrous, D. N.; Exercise-induced promotion of hippocampal cell proliferation requires β-endorphin. *The FASEB Journal,* Vol. 22 July 2008.

Moningka, Natasha C.; Sindler, Amy L.; Muller-Delp, Judy M.; Baylis, Chris; Twelve weeks of treadmill exercise does not alter age-dependent chronic kidney disease in the Fisher 344 male rat. *J Physiol* 589.24, 2011.

Morris J. N., Heady J. A., Raffle P. A. et al. Coronary heart-disease and physical activity of work. *Lancet* 1953; 265:1111-20.

Myers J., Kaykha A., George S. et al. Fitness versus physical activity patterns in predicting mortality in men. *Am J Med* 2004;117:912-8.

Noireaud, Jacques; Andriantsitohaina, Ramaroson. Recent Insights in the Paracrine Modulation of Cardiomyocyte Contractility by Cardiac Endothelial Cells. *Bio Med Research International.* Vol. 2014, Article ID 923805.

Paffenbarger R. S. Jr., Brand R. J., Sholtz R. I. et al. Energy expenditure, cigarette smoking, and blood pressure level as related to death from specific diseases. *Am J Epidemiol* 1978; 108:12-8.

Paffenbarger R. S. Jr., Hyde R. T. Wing A. L. Hsieh C. C. Physical activity, all-cause mortality, and longevity of college alumni. *N Engl J Med.* 1986; 314:605-613.

Pal S., Radavelli-Bagatini S., Ho S. Potential benefits of exercise on blood pressure and vascular function. *J Am Soc Hypertens.* 2013 Nov-Dec; 7(6): 494-506.

Pedersen B. K. Exercise-induced myokines and their role in chronic diseases. *Brain Behav Immun.* 2011 Jul; 25(5):811-6.

Pedersen B. K. The anti-inflammatory effect of exercise: its role in diabetes and cardiovascular disease control. *Essays Biochem.* 2006; 42:105-17.

Pinto A., di Raimondo D., Tuttolomondo A., Buttà C., Milio G., Licata G. Effects of physical exercise on inflammatory markers of atherosclerosis. *Curr Pharm Des.* 2012; 18(28):4326-49.

Prasad D. S., Das B. C. Physical inactivity: a cardiovascular risk factor. *Indian J Med Sci.* 2009 Jan; 63(1):33-42.

Roxburgh B. H., Nolan P. B., Weatherwax R. M., Dalleck L. C. Is moderate intensity exercise training combined with high intensity interval training more effective at improving cardiorespiratory fitness than moderate intensity exercise training alone? *J Sports Sci Med.* 2014 Sep 1;13(3):702-7. eCollection 2014 Sep.

Ryan, A. S.; Ge, S.; Blumenthal, J. B.; Serra, M. C.; Prior, S. J.; Goldberg, A. P. Aerobic exercise and weight loss reduce vascular markers of inflammation and improve insulin sensitivity in obese women. *Journal of American Geriatric Society,* v. 62(4), p. 607-614, 2014.

Rowley, Nicola J.; Dawson, Ellen A.; Birk, Gurpreet K.; Cable, N. Timothy; George, Keith; Whyte, Greg; Thijssen, Dick H. J.; Green, Daniel J.; Exercise and arterial adaptation in humans: uncoupling localized and systemic effects. *J Appl Physiol,* 2011.

Schöllhorn W. I., Beckmann H., Davids K. Exploiting system fluctuations. Differential training in physical prevention and rehabilitation programs for health and exercise. *Medicina* (Kaunas). 2010; 46(6):365-73.

Skrypnik, D.; Bogdański, P.; Madry, E.; Pupek-Musialik, D.; Walkowiak, J. Effect of physical exercise on endothelial function, indicators of inflammation and oxidative stress. *Polski Merkuriusz Lekarski,* v. 36(212), p. 117-121, 2014.

Slattery, K. M.; Dascombe, B.; Wallace, L. K.; Bentley, D. J.; Coutts, A. J. Effect of N-acetylcysteine on Cycling Performance after Intensified Training. *Medical Science and Sports Exercise,* v. 46(6), p. 1114-1123, 2014.

Silva I. C. M., Mostarda C., Moreira E. D., Silva K. A. S., Santos F., Angelis K., Farah V. M. A., Irigoyen M. C.; Preventive role of exercise training in autonomic, hemodynamic, and metabolic parameters in rats under high risk of metabolic syndrome development. *J Appl Physiol.,* 114: 786–791, 2013.

Smuder, A. J.; Kavazis, A. N.; Min, K.; Powers, S. K.; Exercise protects against doxorubicin-induced markers of autophagy signaling in skeletal muscle. *Journal of Applied Physiology,* 2011.

Teodoro, B. G.; Moreira, O. C.; Peluzio, M. C. G.; Natali, A. J.; *Resposta das citocinas ao exercício físico.* http://www.efdeportes.com/Revista Digital-Buenos Aires - Ano 15 - N° 144 - 2010.

Terra, Rodrigo; Silva, Sílvia Amaral Gonçalves da; Pinto, Verônica Salerno; Dutra, Patrícia Maria Lourenço. Efeito do Exercício no Sistema Imune: Resposta, Adaptação E Sinalização Celular. *Rev Bras Med Esporte* - Vol. 18, No 3. Mai/Jun, 2012.

Teixeira-Lemos E., Nunes S., Teixeira F., Reis F. Regular physical exercise training assists in preventing type 2 diabetes development: focus on its antioxidant and anti-inflammatory properties. *Cardiovasc Diabetol.* 2011 Jan 28; 10:12. doi: 10.1186/1475-2840-10-12.

U. S. Department of Health and Human Services. *Physical Activity and Health: A Report of the Surgeon General.* Atlanta, GA: U.S. Department of Health and Human Services, Centers for Disease Control and Prevention, National Center for Chronic Disease Prevention and Health Promotion. 1996.

Umpierre D., Stein R. Hemodynamic and vascular effects of resistance training: implications for cardiovascular disease. *Arq Bras Cardiol* 2007; 89:233-9.

Whyte J. J., Laughlin M. H. The effects of acute and chronic exercise on the vasculature. *Acta Physiol* (Oxf). 2010 Aug; 199(4):441-50. doi: 10.1111/j. 1748-1716.2010.02127.x. Epub 2010 Mar 26.

Warburton D. E., Gledhill N., Quinneya. Musculoskeletal fitness and health. *Can J Appl Physiol* 2001; 26:217-37.

Williams P. T. Physical fitness and activity as separate heart disease risk factors: a meta-analysis. *Med Sci Sports Exerc* 2001;33:754-61.

Wycherley Thomas Philip; Clifton, Peter Marshall; Noakes, Manny; Brinkworth, Grant David; Weight loss on a structured hypocaloric diet with or without exercise improves emotional distress and quality of life in overweight and obese patients with type 2 diabetes. *J Diabetes Invest,* Vol. 5, 2014.

Zelber-Sagi Shira, Buch Assaf, Yeshua Hanny, Vaisman Nahum, Webb Muriel, Harari Gil, Kis Ofer, Fliss-Isakov Naomi, Izkhakov Elena, Halpern Zamir, Santo Erwin, OREN Ran, SHIBOLET Oren. Effect of resistance training on non-alcoholic fatty-liver disease a randomized-clinical trial. *World J Gastroenterol,* 2014.

In: Exercise Training
Editor: Lucy Dukes

ISBN: 978-1-63463-501-1

Chapter 4

MELATONIN, EXERCISE TRAINING AND BENEFITS: A REVIEW

J. S. Silva-Junior*[1], *C. Mendes*[1], *R. A. Matos*[1], *L. C. Motta-Teixeira*[1], *J. Andrade-Silva*[1], *F. G. Amaral*[2] *and J. Cipolla-Neto*[1]

[1]Neurobiology Lab, Department of Physiology and Biophysics, Institute of Biomedical Sciences, University of São Paulo, São Paulo, Brazil

[2]Department of Physiology, UNIFESP, São Paulo, Brazil

ABSTRACT

The pineal gland is responsible for the synthesis and secretion of the hormone melatonin, which, in turn, participates in the temporal organization of biological rhythms acting as a mediator between the light / dark cycle and regulatory physiological processes, including the regulation of the cardiovascular system, immune system and, among others, the energy metabolism, influencing the secretion and action of insulin and increasing the thermogenic capacity of brown adipose tissue and the browning process. Moreover, melatonin presents powerful antioxidant, neuroprotective and neurogenic actions. The available data shows that melatonin is essential for adipose and muscle tissues

* Corresponding author: cipolla@icb.usp.br
J.S.Silva-Junior and C. Mendes, contributed equally for this publication

metabolic adaptations to aerobic training. On the other hand, exercise training plays a key role in the control of glycemia, blood pressure, adult neurogenesis and browning of white adipose tissue. The reduction of melatonin production that occurs during aging, in diabetes, during shift-work or at illuminated environments during the night, not only impairs the metabolic benefits of exercise training but also induces several metabolic disorders such as insulin resistance, glucose intolerance, obesity and cardiovascular disturbances. Considering the available scientific evidence, clinicians may consider melatonin replacement or supplementation in certain situations, as the ones mentioned above, as an additional therapeutic tool in order to favor all the beneficial effects of the physical training.

INTRODUCTION

Melatonin is a very ancient molecule being present in almost all living organisms. It is an indolamine known for its amphiphilic characteristic that allows it to be found in all compartments of the body and of the cell. This molecule also presents a high antioxidant capacity, being one of the most important natural antioxidants in the body (Tan et al., 2002).

In mammals, the hormone melatonin is produced by the pineal gland that is under control of the circadian clock and synchronized to the daily illumination cycle typical of the day and night. This control is such that melatonin is produced exclusively at night and the duration of its daily plasma profile varies in accordance to the duration of the night in different seasons (Afeche et al., 2008). As a consequence, the pineal gland is considered a photoneuroendocrine transducer and melatonin is known as a mediator between the cyclic environmental light-dark cycle and the physiological rhythmic (circadian and seasonal) adaptive processes associated to vital functions such as reproduction (Goldman, 2001), cardiovascular system (McKinley et al., 1990), rest-activity and sleep-wake cycles (Armstrong, 1989), immune responses (Fraschini et al., 1990), energy metabolism (Cipolla-Neto et al., 2014), among others.

Melatonin, Energy Metabolism and the Physiological Adaptation to Physical Exercise Training

One of the main functions of melatonin is to regulate insulin secretion and peripheral and central insulin actions (Cipolla-Neto et al., 2014; Zanuto et al., 2013; Lima et al., 1998). The absence of melatonin or its reduction, as observed in aging, promotes insulin resistance and glucose intolerance in addition to an impairment of pancreatic insulin secretion. Moreover, melatonin is the key mediator molecule for the integration between the cyclic environment and the circadian and seasonal distribution of physiological and behavioral processes associated to energy balance and body weight regulation (Cipolla-Neto et al., 2014). Melatonin regulates energy intake (feeding) (Montano et al., 2010), energy flow to and from storage sites (Nogueira et al, 2011) and energy expenditure, regulating the activity and trophism of brown adipose tissue and the browning processes of the white adipose tissue (Jiménez-Aranda et al., 2013; Ralph, 1984; Tan et al., 2011).

Pinealectomized animals (Borges-Silva et al., 2007; Borges-Silva et al., 2005a; Borges-Silva et al., 2005b; Lopes et al., unpublished observations), showing an absence of circulating melatonin, fail to develop the adaptive metabolic capacity induced by exercise training (insulin-stimulated glucose uptake, conversion of d- [U-^{14}C]-glucose, l- [U-^{14}C]-lactate, [2-^{14}C]-acetate and [1-^{14}C]-palmitate into $^{14}CO_2$; lipolysis, lipogenesis, hexokinase, pyruvate kinase, lactate dehydrogenase, citrate synthase and malic enzyme activities, hepatic and muscular glycogen content) and therefore do not present the same performance of the control animals. On the other hand, the replacement therapy with melatonin, restore all the metabolic and behavioral adaptations to the physical training, improving the physical performance to the level of the control group.

As far as the effects of exercise training on the daily production of melatonin is concerned, the available data in humans are contradictory. Although some studies show an increase in melatonin plasma levels due to exercise (Buxton et al., 1997; Carr et al., 1981; Skrinar et al., 1989; Theron et al., 1984) other studies suggest a decrease (Monteleone et al., 1992; Monteleone et al., 1990) or no alterations (Elias et al., 1993; Miyazaki et al., 2001; Yaga et al., 1993).

MELATONIN AND THE ADAPTATION OF THE AGING ORGANISM TO PHYSICAL TRAINING

As the physiological process of aging takes place, the biosynthesis of melatonin by the pineal gland decreases (Karasek, 2004; Pang et al., 1990) leading to a deterioration of many circadian rhythms and several physiological processes, such as the sleep / wake cycle, energy metabolism, body temperature, alertness and secretion of many hormones. Furthermore, due to its antioxidative property, the reduction in melatonin production related to aging can lead to accumulation of free radicals, reflecting not only in aging itself, but also in several age-related diseases. As melatonin also presents immunostimulatory properties, the relative immunosuppression due to the reduction in melatonin production might be involved in the acceleration of aging processes (Ginaldi et al., 1999a; Ginaldi et al., 1999b; Ginaldi et al., 1999c; Maestroni, 2001). From the energy metabolism point of view, the decrease in circulating melatonin levels can lead to a variety of physiological changes associated with aging (Rasmussen et al., 1999), such as an increase in adiposity, especially visceral, and in plasma levels of insulin and leptin (Bjorntorp, 1995), glucose intolerance, insulin resistance, diabetes, and dyslipidemia that associated to the hypertension can characterize the classical metabolic syndrome (Bodkin et al., 1996; Buemann and Tremblay, 1996; Zanuto et al., 2013).

Mendes et al., (2013) demonstrated that the reduced levels of circulating melatonin, impairs the physiological adaptations induced by exercise training in aged rats. Moreover, melatonin supplementation to the aging animals was highly efficient to reduce body weight and to improve glucose tolerance, physical capacity, citrate synthase activity, hepatic and muscular glycogen content, and also to increase the expression of proteins related to the insulin signaling pathway both in the liver and in skeletal muscle, improving considerably the physical performance. It should be emphasized that, in the same context, Zanuto et al., (2013) demonstrated that 8 weeks of melatonin supplementation to aged rats was able to restore insulin signaling to the levels of young animals in both central and peripheral tissues (muscle, adipose tissue, and liver). This improvement in insulin signaling preceded by 4 weeks the weight reduction observed in the same animals.

MELATONIN, EXERCISE TRAINING AND DIABETES

Diabetes mellitus is a complex and primary metabolic disorder. It is characterized by hyperglycemia resulting from progressive loss of insulin action or secretion (Zimmet et al., 2001). Researchers indicate that the estimated number of adults living with diabetes increased to 382 million, representing 8.3% of the population worldwide. This number will increase to 592 million in less than 25 years from now (International Diabetes Federation, 2013).

The classic therapeutical strategies in combination with non-pharmacological therapies represent a tool in the prevention and control of diabetes mellitus. Aerobic exercise training improves insulin sensitivity through multiple factors, as increased muscle mass, increased blood flow and activation of glucose transport (Koivisto et al., 1986).

Through an independent action of insulin that involves muscle contraction, physical exercise plays a key role in the control of blood sugar levels by stimulating glucose uptake (DeFronzo et al., 1987; Lund et al., 1995; Wallberg-Henriksson and Holloszy, 1984). Aerobic exercise has been considered the most suitable one to improve insulin sensitivity, but it is not clear how factors such as intensity, duration or frequency are involved in the effects (Kang et al., 1996).

Evidences show that experimental diabetes induced by alloxan or streptozotocin (STZ) significantly decreases pineal and plasma melatonin levels in rats (Amaral et al., 2014; Champney et al., 1986; Pang et al., 1985). In STZ-induced diabetic rats, the significant decrease in the synthesis of pineal melatonin is probably caused by the hyperglycemia, with decreased expression of the beta adrenergic receptor, reduced cAMP levels, and impaired protein expression and activity of AANAT in the pineal (Amaral et al., 2014). The same inverse correlation between hyperglycemia and melatonin production was seen in type 1-diabetes patients (Amaral et al., 2014).

Considering, as mentioned above, that supplementation with melatonin improves insulin secretion and signaling and it is essential to promote the metabolic adaptation to physical training (DeOliveira et al., 2012; Mendes et al., 2013), the therapeutic association of melatonin supplementation should be considered in addition to the exercise prescription to diabetes patients (Houmard et al., 2004).

MELATONIN, PHYSICAL TRAINING AND ADULT NEUROGENESIS

Adult neurogenesis (AN) is the production of new neurons in adult brain. The term neurogenesis refers to a complex process that begins with the proliferation of progenitor cells, followed by differentiation /determination of neuronal phenotype maturation, morphological and physiological development of the characteristics of neuronal functioning, and ends up with the existence of a new functional neuron that is integrated to the existing networks (Kempermann, 2011).

In the adult mammalian brain, at least two regions of the central nervous system are canonically classified as neurogenic niches, the subventricular zone of the lateral ventricles (SVZ) and the subgranular zone of the dentate gyrus of the hippocampus (SGZ) (Abrous et al., 2005; Ehninger and Kempermann, 2008; Gage et al., 1998; Gould et al., 1999). The AN process is part of different biological processes such as learning, memory, and neuropsychiatric disorders (Noonan et al., 2010; Sahay and Hen, 2008; Snyder et al., 2011).

Intrinsic and extrinsic dynamic factors may affect different stages of the neurogenesis process, including expansion (proliferation), differentiation (i.e. neuronal versus glial) and survival. For example, the aging process and the sleep deprivation lead to a drastic reduction of cell proliferation in SGZ and SVZ (Kuhn et al., 1996; Rossi et al., 2006). Another important negative regulator of adult neurogenesis is the inflammation induced by injury, neurodegenerative diseases and irradiation (Carpentier and Palmer, 2009).

There is evidence that sleep may contribute to hippocampal function by inducing/enhancing the process of neurogenesis. Sleep deprivation for 96 hours reduces proliferation and neurogenesis in adult rats (Guzman-Marin et al., 2005; Ramirez-Rodriguez et al., 2009) and sleep fragmentation can also damage plastic processes in the brain (Mueller et al., 2011). This modulation occurs through mechanisms independent of glucocorticoids, a negative modulator of neurogenesis (Mueller et al., 2011). Changes in the circadian rhythm can also affect neurogenesis, it is known that the rate of cell proliferation fluctuates with the light–dark cycle (Gilhooley et al., 2011; Guzman-Marin et al., 2007; Tamai et al., 2008). Moreover, the levels of hormones and growth factors influence the proliferation and differentiation of neural progenitor cells under physiological and pathological conditions (Sotthibundhu et al., 2010).

It has been recently suggested that melatonin can contribute to the process of neurogenesis (Manda and Reiter, 2010; Ramirez-Rodriguez et al., 2011; Ramirez-Rodriguez et al., 2009; Rennie et al., 2009). It is known that the administration of exogenous melatonin does not increase the rate of proliferation of neural progenitor cells even with 3 weeks of treatment (Jang et al., 2010; Sompol et al., 2011) however, it modulates the survival of cells that have undergone the process of proliferation (Ramirez-Rodriguez et al., 2011). The modulation that melatonin exerts in the proliferation, differentiation and survival of neural progenitor cells occurs via melatonin-membrane receptors (MT1 and MT2), since the use of the melatonin-receptor antagonist luzindol inhibits the beneficial effects (Kong et al., 2008; Moriya et al., 2007; Sotthibundhu et al., 2010). In addition, melatonin increases the maturation of dendrites and the complexity of newly generated neurons to facilitate their incorporation into existing neural circuits, an important factor in the process of survival (Benítez-King, 2006). The drug agomelatine, that is a synthetic melatonin-receptor agonist, leads to an increase in the proportion of hippocampal granular mature neurons and neurite growth, suggesting an acceleration of the process of maturation. The influence of agomelatine in the maturation and survival of the cell is accompanied by a selective increase in the levels of BDNF (neurotrophic factor derived from the brain) that plays a role in the control of neuronal proliferation and survival (Soumier et al., 2009).

A number of studies have reported physical activity as one of the strongest inducers of neurogenesis in the dentate gyrus of young, adult and aged animals (Fabel and Kempermann, 2008; Kannangara et al., 2011; Kim et al., 2007; Kohman et al., 2012; Kronenberg et al., 2006; Kronenberg et al., 2003; Van Praag et al., 1999). The effects of physical exercise on the dentate gyrus of rodents can be observed 24 hours after the first training session. However, the detection of more pronounced effects occurs after 3 days of physical activity (Ferreira et al., 2011; Van Praag et al., 1999). Physical activity has a pro-proliferative effect acting primarily on amplifying progenitor cells (type II) in the hippocampus (Kronenberg et al., 2003; Steiner et al., 2008). There is a non-independent apparent effect on subsequent stages of neuronal development, involving the promotion of survival. Even when the effect of proliferation returns to baseline levels, the population of cells that are positive for DCX (protein expressed in microtubules in young neurons) continues to increase (Kronenberg et al., 2003).

Therefore, exercise seems to mobilize a cascade of molecular events that culminates in the formation of new neurons in the hippocampal region, with consequent increase in synaptic plasticity and improvement of the processes of learning and memory (Cotman and Berchtold, 2007).

As melatonin acts as a positive modulator of differentiation, maturation and survival of new cells through the activation of a variety of mechanisms (membrane receptors, free radical scavenger, or as a modulator of the cytoskeleton reorganization), it is possible that physical exercise associated with melatonin supplementation or replacement (to specific groups) may promote not only neurogenesis, but also the survival and recruitment of these new neurons and their integration with hippocampal circuits. Recently, Liu et al., (2013) demonstrated that the cell proliferation induced by 12 days of voluntary running is not influenced by treatment with oral melatonin during the same period. However, melatonin treatment facilitated cell survival and neurogenesis induced by exercise.

Although these results suggest a new treatment prospect, additional studies are required to test the clinical efficacy of melatonin supplementation associated with physical activity and plasticity of the nervous system.

Conclusion

Melatonin, due to its ancient origin and prevalence in nature, is a powerful antioxidant and a critical hormone responsible for the adequate adaptation of the vertebrate organism to the cyclic daily and seasonal environment. Melatonin is important for the proper physiological metabolic adaptations necessary for the support of the circadian activity-feeding/rest-fasting behavioral cycle. The absence or reduction in melatonin production, as in aging and diabetes, leads to metabolic disorders and chronodisruption that impairs all the beneficial effects of the physical training, making melatonin replacement or supplementation a tool to be considered.

References

Abrous DN, Koehl M, Le Moal M. Adult neurogenesis: from precursors to network and physiology. *Physiol. Rev.*, 2005 85,523–69.

Afeche SC, Amaral FG, Villela DCM, Abrahão MV, Peres R, Cipolla-Neto, J. Melatonin and the pineal gland. In: Romano E, De Luca S. In: New

Research on Neurosecretory Systems. US: Nova Science Publishers; 2008. 151 – 177.

Amaral FG, Turati AO, Barone M, Scialfa JH, Do Carmo Buonfiglio D, Peres R, Peliciari-Garcia RA, Afeche SC, Lima L, Bordin S, Reiter RJ, Menna-Barreto L, Cipolla-Neto J. Melatonin synthesis impairment as a new deleterious outcome of diabetes-derived hyperglycemia. *J. Pineal Res.,* 2014 57,67–79.

Armstrong SM. Melatonin and circadian control in mammals. *Experientia.,* 1989 45,932–8.

Benítez-King G. Melatonin as a cytoskeletal modulator: Implications for cell physiology and disease. *J. Pineal Res.*, 2006 40(1), 1–9.

Bjorntorp P. Neuroendocrine aging. *J. Intern. Med.*, 1995 238, 401–4.

Bodkin NL, Nicolson M, Ortmeyer HK, Hansen BC. Hyperleptinemia: relationship to adiposity and insulin resistance in the spontaneously obese rhesus monkey. *Horm. Metab. Res.*, 1996 28, 674–8.

Borges-Silva CN, Alonso-Vale MIC, Franzói-De-Moraes SM, Takada J, Peres SB, Andreotti S, Skorupa AL, Cipolla-Neto J, Pithon-Curi TC, Lima FB. Pinealectomy impairs adipose tissue adaptability to exercise in rats. *J. Pineal Res.*, 2005a 38, 278–83.

Borges-Silva CN, Fonseca-Alaniz MH, Alonso-Vale MI, Takada J, Andreotti S, Peres SB, Cipolla-Neto J, Pithon-Curi TC, Lima FB. Reduced lipolysis and increased lipogenesis in adipose tissue from pinealectomized rats adapted to training. *J. Pineal Res*, 2005b 39(2), 178-84.

Borges-Silva CN, Takada J, Alonso-Vale MIC, Peres SB, Fonseca-Alaniz MH, Andreotti S, Cipolla-Neto J, Pithon-Curi TC, Lima FB. Pinealectomy reduces hepatic and muscular glycogen content and attenuates aerobic power adaptability in trained rats. *J. Pineal Res.*, 2007 43, 96–103.

Buemann B, Tremblay A. Effects of exercise training on abdominal obesity and related metabolic complications. *Sport. Med.*, 1996 21, 191–212.

Buxton OM, L'Hermite-Balériaux M, Hirschfeld U, Cauter E. Acute and delayed effects of exercise on human melatonin secretion. *J. Biol. Rhythms,* 1997 12, 568–74.

Carpentier PA, Palmer TD. Immune Influence on Adult Neural Stem Cell Regulation and Function. *Neuron,* 2009 64(1), 79–92.

Carr DB, Reppert SM, Bullen B, Skrinar G, Beitins I, Arnold M, Rosenblatt M, McArthut JW. Plasma melatonin increases during exercise in women. *J. Clin. Endocrinol. Metab.*, 1981 53, 224–6.

Champney TH, Holtorf AP, Craft CM, Reiter RJ. Hormonal modulation of pineal melatonin synthesis in rats and Syrian hamsters: effects of streptozotocin-induced diabetes and insulin injections. *Comp. Biochem. Physiol. A. Comp. Physiol.*, 1986 83, 391–5.

Cipolla-Neto J, Amaral FG, Afeche SC, Tan DX, Reiter RJ. Melatonin, energy metabolism, and obesity: A review. *J. Pineal Res.,* 2014 56, 371–81.

Cotman CW, Berchtold NC. Physical activity and the maintenance of cognition: Learning from animal models. *Alzheimer's Dement.*, 2007 3(2 Suppl), S30-7.

DeFronzo RA, Sherwin RS, Kraemer N. Effect of physical training on insulin action in obesity. *Diabetes,* 1987 36, 1379–85.

DeOliveira AC, Andreotti S, Da T, Torres-Leal FL, De Proença ARG, Campaña AB, et al., Metabolic disorders and adipose tissue insulin responsiveness in neonatally STZ-induced diabetic rats are improved by long-term melatonin treatment. *Endocrinology,* 2012 153, 2178–88.

Ehninger D, Kempermann G. Neurogenesis in the adult hippocampus. *Cell Tissue Res.,* 2008 331(1), 243–50.

Elias AN, Wilson AF, Pandian MR, Rojas FJ, Kayaleh R, Stone SC, James N. Melatonin and gonadotropin secretion after acute exercise in physically active males. *Eur. J. Appl. Physiol. Occup. Physiol.*, 1993 66(4), 357–61.

Fabel K, Kempermann G. Physical activity and the regulation of neurogenesis in the adult and aging brain. *Neuromolecular M*ed., 2008 10, 59–66.

Ferreira AFB, Real CC, Rodrigues AC, Alves AS, Britto LRG. Short-term, moderate exercise is capable of inducing structural, bdnf-independent hippocampal plasticity. *Brain Res.*, 2011 1425, 111–22.

Fraschini F, Scaglione F, Franco P, Demartini G, Lucini V, Stankov B. Melatonin and immunity. *Acta Oncol.*, 1990 29(6), 775-6.

Gage FH, Kempermann G, Palmer TD, Peterson DA, Ray J. Multipotent progenitor cells in the adult dentate gyrus. *J. Neurobiol.*, 1998 36, 249–66.

Gilhooley MJ, Pinnock SB, Herbert J. Rhythmic expression of per1 in the dentate gyrus is suppressed by corticosterone: Implications for neurogenesis. *Neurosci. Lett.*, 2011 489, 177–81.

Ginaldi L, De Martinis M, D'Ostilio A, Marini L, Loreto MF, Corsi MP, Quaglino D. The immune system in the elderly: I. Specific humoral immunity. *Immunol. Res.*, 1999a 20, 101–8.

Ginaldi L, De Martinis M, D'Ostilio A, Marini L, Loreto MF, Martorelli V, Quaglino D. The immune system in the elderly: II. Specific cellular immunity. *Immunol. Res.*, 1999b 20, 109–15.

Ginaldi L, De Martinis M, D'Ostilio A, Marini L, Loreto MF, Quaglino D. The immune system in the elderly: III. Innate immunity. *Immunol. Res.,* 1999c 20, 117–26.

Goldman BD. Mammalian photoperiodic system: formal properties and neuroendocrine mechanisms of photoperiodic time measurement. *J. Biol. Rhythms,* 2001 16, 283–301.

Gould E, Reeves AJ, Fallah M, Tanapat P, Gross CG, Fuchs E. Hippocampal neurogenesis in adult Old World primates. *Proc. Natl. Acad. Sci. U. S. A.*, 1999 96, 5263–7.

Guzman-Marin R, Suntsova N, Methippara M, Greiffenstein R, Szymusiak R, McGinty D. Sleep deprivation suppresses neurogenesis in the adult hippocampus of rats. *Eur. J. Neurosci.*, 2005 22, 2111–6.

Guzman-Marin R, Suntsova N, Bashir T, Szymusiak R, McGinty D. Cell proliferation in the dentate gyrus of the adult rat fluctuates with the light-dark cycle. *Neurosci. Lett.*, 2007 422, 198–201.

Houmard JA, Tanner CJ, Slentz CA, Duscha BD, McCartney JS, Kraus WE. Effect of the volume and intensity of exercise training on insulin sensitivity. *J. Appl. Physiol.,* 2004 96(1), 101–6.

International Diabetes Federation. Diabetes Atlas. Sixth Edition. 2013.

Jang S-W, Liu X, Pradoldej S, Tosini G, Chang Q, Iuvone PM, Ye K. N-acetylserotonin activates TrkB receptor in a circadian rhythm. *Proc. Natl. Acad. Sci. U. S. A.,* 2010 107, 3876–81.

Jiménez-Aranda A, Fernández-Vázquez G, Campos D, Tassi M, Velasco-Perez L, Tan DX, Reiter RJ, Agil A. Melatonin induces browning of inguinal white adipose tissue in Zucker diabetic fatty rats. *J. Pineal Res.,* 2013 55, 416–23.

Kang J, Robertson RJ, Hagberg JM, Kelley DE, Goss FL, DaSilva SG, Suminski RR, Utter AC. Effect of exercise intensity on glucose and insulin metabolism in obese individuals and obese NIDDM patients. *Diabetes Care.*, 1996 19, 341–9.

Kannangara TS, Lucero MJ, Gil-Mohapel J, Drapala RJ, Simpson JM, Christie BR, van Praag H. Running reduces stress and enhances cell genesis in aged mice. *Neurobiol. Aging*, 2011 32, 2279–86.

Karasek M. Melatonin, human aging, and age-related diseases. *Exp. Gerontol.,* 2004 39(11-12), 1723–9.

Kempermann G. Adult Neurogenesis 2: Stem Cells and Neuronal Development in the Adult Brain. Oxford University: Press; 2011.

Kim H, Lee S-H, Kim S-S, Yoo J-H, Kim C-J. The influence of maternal treadmill running during pregnancy on short-term memory and hippocampal cell survival in rat pups. *Int. J. Dev. Neurosci.*, 2007 25(4), 243–9.

Kohman RA, DeYoung EK, Bhattacharya TK, Peterson LN, Rhodes JS. Wheel running attenuates microglia proliferation and increases expression of a proneurogenic phenotype in the hippocampus of aged mice. *Brain. Behav. Immun.*, 2012 26, 803–10.

Koivisto VA, Yki-Järvinen H, DeFronzo RA. Physical training and insulin sensitivity. *Diabetes. Metab. Rev.*, 1986 1, 445–81.

Kong X, Li X, Cai Z, Yang N, Liu Y, Shu J, Pan L, Zuo P. Melatonin regulates the viability and differentiation of rat midbrain neural stem cells. *Cell. Mol. Neurobiol.*, 2008 28, 569–79.

Kronenberg G, Reuter K, Steiner B, Brandt MD, Jessberger S, Yamaguchi M, Kempermann G. Subpopulations of proliferating cells of the adult hippocampus respond differently to physiologic neurogenic stimuli. *J. Comp. Neurol.*, 2003 467(4), 455–63.

Kronenberg G, Bick-Sander a, Bunk E, Wolf C, Ehninger D, Kempermann G. Physical exercise prevents age-related decline in precursor cell activity in the mouse dentate gyrus. *Neurobiol. Aging*, 2006 27, 1505–13.

Kuhn HG, Dickinson-Anson H, Gage FH. Neurogenesis in the dentate gyrus of the adult rat: age-related decrease of neuronal progenitor proliferation. *J. Neurosci.*, 1996 16, 2027–33.

Lima FB, Machado UF, Bartol I, Seraphim PM, Sumida DH, Moraes SM, Hell NS, Okamoto MM, Saad MJ, Carvalho CR, Cipolla-Neto J. Pinealectomy causes glucose intolerance and decreases adipose cell responsiveness to insulin in rats. *Am. J. Physiol.*, 1998 275(6 Pt1), E934-41.

Liu J, Somera-Molina KC, Hudson RL, Dubocovich ML. Melatonin potentiates running wheel-induced neurogenesis in the dentate gyrus of adult C3H/HeN mice hippocampus. *J. Pineal Res.*, 2013 54, 222–31.

Lund S, Holman GD, Schmitz O, Pedersen O. Contraction stimulates translocation of glucose transporter GLUT4 in skeletal muscle through a mechanism distinct from that of insulin. *Proc. Natl. Acad. Sci. U. S. A.*, 1995 92, 5817–21.

Maestroni GJ. The immunotherapeutic potential of melatonin. *Expert Opin. Investig. Drugs.*, 2001 10, 467–76.

Manda K, Reiter RJ. Melatonin maintains adult hippocampal neurogenesis and cognitive functions after irradiation. *Prog. Neurobiol.*, 2010 90(1), 60–8.

McKinley MJ, McAllen RM, Mendelsohn FAO, Allen AM, Chai SY, Oldfield BJ. Circumventricular organs - neuroendocrine interfaces between the brain and the hemal milieu. *Front. Neuroendocrinol.*, 1990 11, 91–127.

Mendes C, Lopes AMDS, Do Amaral FG, Peliciari-Garcia RA, Turati ADO, Hirabara SM, Scialfa JH, Cipolla-Neto J. Adaptations of the aging animal to exercise: Role of daily supplementation with melatonin. *J. Pineal Res.,* 2013 55, 229–39.

Miyazaki T, Hashimoto S, Masubuchi S, Honma S, Honma KI. Phase-advance shifts of human circadian pacemaker are accelerated by daytime physical exercise. *Am. J. Physiol. Regul. Integr. Comp. Physiol.*, 2001 281, R197–R205.

Montano ME, Molpeceres V, Mauriz JL, Garzo E, Cruz IBM, González P, Barrio JP. Effect of melatonin supplementation on food and water intake in streptozotocin-diabetic and non-diabetic male Wistar rats. *Nutr. Hosp.,* 2010 25(6), 931–8.

Monteleone P, Maj M, Fusco M, Orazzo C, Kemali D. Physical exercise at night blunts the nocturnal increase of plasma melatonin levels in healthy humans. *Life Sci.*, 1990 47, 1989–95.

Monteleone P, Maj M, Fuschino A, Kemali D. Physical stress in the middle of the dark phase does not affect light -depressed plasma melatonin levels in humans. *Neuroendocrinology*, 1992 55, 367–71.

Moriya T, Horie N, Mitome M, Shinohara K. Melatonin influences the proliferative and differentiative activity of neural stem cells. J. *Pineal Res.*, 2007 42, 411–8.

Mueller AD, Mear RJ, Mistlberger RE. Inhibition of hippocampal neurogenesis by sleep deprivation is independent of circadian disruption and melatonin suppression. *Neuroscience,* 2011 193, 170–81.

Nogueira TC, Lellis-Santos C, Jesus DS, Taneda M, Rodrigues SC, Amaral FG, Lopes AM, Cipolla-Neto J, Bordin S, Anhê GF. Absence of melatonin induces night-time hepatic insulin resistance and increased gluconeogenesis due to stimulation of nocturnal unfolded protein protein response. *Endocrinology,* 2011 152(4), 1253-63.

Noonan MA, Bulin SE, Fuller DC, Eisch AJ. Reduction of adult hippocampal neurogenesis confers vulnerability in an animal model of cocaine addiction. *J. Neurosci.*, 2010 30, 304–15.

Pang SF, Tang F, Tang PL. Alloxan-induced diabetes and the pineal gland: differential effects on the levels of pineal N-acetylserotonin, pineal melatonin, and serum melatonin. *J. Pineal Res.*, 1985 2, 79–85.

Pang SF, Tsang CW, Hong GX, Yip PCY, Tang PL, Brown GM. Fluctuation of blood melatonin concentrations with age: Result of changes in pineal melatonin secretion, body growth, and aging. *J. Pineal Res.*, 1990 8, 179–92.

Ralph CL. Pineal bodies and thermorregulation. In: *Reiter J. The pineal gland.* New York: Raven; 1984; 193-220.

Ramirez-Rodriguez G, Klempin F, Babu H, Benitez-King G, Kempermann G. Melatonin Modulates Cell Survival of New Neurons in the Hippocampus of Adult Mice. *Neuropsychopharmacology,* 2009 34, 2180–91.

Ramirez-Rodriguez G, Ortíz-Lõpez L, Domínguez-Alonso A, Benítez-King GA, Kempermann G. Chronic treatment with melatonin stimulates dendrite maturation and complexity in adult hippocampal neurogenesis of mice. *J. Pineal Res.*, 2011 50, 29–37.

Rasmussen DD, Boldt BM, Wilkinson CW, Yellon SM, Matsumoto AM. Daily melatonin administration at middle age suppresses male rat visceral fat, plasma leptin, and plasma insulin to youthful levels. *Endocrinology,* 1999 140, 1009–12.

Rennie K, De Butte M, Pappas BA. Melatonin promotes neurogenesis in dentate gyrus in the pinealectomized rat. *J. Pineal Res.*, 2009 47, 313–7.

Rossi C, Angelucci A, Costantin L, Braschi C, Mazzantini M, Babbini F, Fabbri ME, Tessarollo L, Berardi N, Caleo M. Brain-derived neurotrophic factor (BDNF) is required for the enhancement of hippocampal neurogenesis following environmental enrichment. *Eur. J. Neurosci.*, 2006 24, 1850–6.

Sahay A, Hen R. Hippocampal neurogenesis and depression. *Novartis Found. Symp.*, 2008 289, 152–160; discussion 160–4, 193–5.

Skrinar GS, Bullen BA, Reppert SM, Peachey SE, Turnbull BA, McArthur JW. Melatonin response to exercise training in women. *J. Pineal Res.,* 1989 7, 185–94.

Snyder JS, Soumier A, Brewer M, Pickel J, Cameron HA. Adult hippocampal neurogenesis buffers stress responses and depressive behaviour. *Nature,* 2011 476, 458–61.

Sompol P, Liu X, Baba K, Paul KN, Tosini G, Iuvone PM, Ye K. N-acetylserotonin promotes hippocampal neuroprogenitor cell proliferation in sleep-deprived mice. *Proc. Natl. Acad. Sci. U. S. A.*, 2011 108(21), 8844–9.

Sotthibundhu A, Phansuwan-Pujito P, Govitrapong P. Melatonin increases proliferation of cultured neural stem cells obtained from adult mouse subventricular zone. *J. Pineal Res.*, 2010 49, 291–300.

Soumier A, Banasr M, Lortet S, Masmejean F, Bernard N, Kerkerian-Le-Goff L, Gabriel C, Millan MJ, Mocaer E, Daszuta A. Mechanisms contributing to the phase-dependent regulation of neurogenesis by the novel antidepressant, agomelatine, in the adult rat hippocampus. *Neuropsychopharmacology,* 2009 34, 2390–403.

Steiner B, Zurborg S, Hörster H, Fabel K, Kempermann G. Differential 24 h responsiveness of Prox1-expressing precursor cells in adult hippocampal neurogenesis to physical activity, environmental enrichment, and kainic acid-induced seizures. *Neuroscience,* 2008 154, 521–9.

Tamai SI, Sanada K, Fukada Y. Time-of-day-dependent enhancement of adult neurogenesis in the hippocampus. *PLoS One*, 2008 3(12), e3835.

Tan DX, Reiter RJ, Manchester LC, Yan M, El-Sawi M, Sainz RM, Mayo JC, Kohen R, Allegra M, Hardeland R. Chemical and physical properties and potential mechanisms: melatonin as a broad spectrum antioxidant and free radical scavenger. *Curr. Top. Med. Chem.,* 2002 2, 181–97.

Tan DX, Manchester LC, Fuentes-Broto L, Paredes SD, Reiter J. Significance and application of melatonin in the regulation of brown adipose tissue metabolism: relation to human obesity. *Obes. Rev*., 2011 12(3), 167-88.

Theron JJ, Oosthuizen JM, Rautenbach MM. Effect of physical exercise on plasma melatonin levels in normal volunteers. S. *Afr. Med. J.* 1984 66, 838–41.

Van Praag H, Christie BR, Sejnowski TJ, Gage FH. Running enhances neurogenesis, learning, and long-term potentiation in mice. *Proc. Natl. Acad. Sci. U. S. A.,* 1999 96, 13427–31.

Wallberg-Henriksson H, Holloszy JO. Contractile activity increases glucose uptake by muscle in severely diabetic rats. *J. Appl. Physiol.*, 1984 57, 1045–9.

Yaga K, Tan DX, Reiter RJ, Manchester LC, Hattori A. Unusual responses of nocturnal pineal melatonin synthesis and secretion to swimming: attempts to define mechanisms. *J. Pineal Res*., 1993 14, 98–103.

Zanuto R, Siqueira-Filho MA, Caperuto LC, Bacurau RFP, Hirata E, Peliciari-Garcia RA, et al., Melatonin improves insulin sensitivity independently of weight loss in old obese rats. J. *Pineal Res*., 2013 55, 156–65.

Zimmet P, Alberti KG, Shaw J. Global and societal implications of the diabetes epidemic. *Nature*, 2001 414, 782–7.

INDEX

C

D

E

F

G

H

I

J

K

L

M

N

O

P

Q

R

S

T

U

V

W